STOP SMOKING NOW!

*Vital Psychodynamics Programmes
to Stop Smoking*

Antony Maurice-Nneke

Originally Published in 2010
NOW, fully revised including the additional entry of a formula to aid success, and ways to confront some major fears that might deter effort to stop smoking.

First Published on Amazon Kendal 2023

British Library Cataloguing in Publication Data

A catalogue record of this book is available from the British Library

ISBN: 9798393663179

Books By the Same Author

2023: Lose Weight Now! Amazon Kendal

2022: Sex and Psychodynamics Psychiatry, Amazon Kendal

2013: Sex and Psychosexuality, Xinjiang Press. China

2003: The Psychodynamics of the Unconscious, Intapsy Publications, London.

2002: Mind Castles, Intapsy Publications, London.

ACKNOWLEDGEMENT

I thank members of my family for their support and, I am particularly grateful to them for their general warmth and kindness during my work on this book.

CONTENTS

ACKNOWLEDGEMENT...v
INTRODUCTION..1
I.1 The Basic Idea of the Mind Technique in This Book.................1
I.2 The Practice Sessions 6
I.3 The Key Points to Remember...6
I.4 Further Useful Secret Programmes in the Book.......................7
I.5 Exude Confidence Always...7
I.6 The Idea of Psycho-cybernetics..9

CHAPTER ONE: ESSENTIAL PRELIMINARY STEPS TO
STOP SMOKING..11
1.1 The Preparatory Exercise 11
1.2 The Fundamental Principles of the Mind Technique...............18
1.3 Key Points to Remember 26
1.4 The Secrets of How the Mind Works....................................26
1.5 Key Points to Remember 33
1.6 Belief as an essential ingredient to Stop Smoking.................34
1.7 You Must Have Total Belief and Faith in Yourself..................35
1.8 Key Points to Remember 36
1.9 How to Eliminate the Negative Power of Self Doubt...............36
1.10 Key Points to Remember 39
1.11 Positive Strategies to Enhance Your Success in Giving up
Smoking 39
1.12 Confront Your Fear to Conquer It......................................40
1.13 How to Deal with the Effects of Stress, Anxiety and
Depression (SAD)...43
1.14 Examining Your Level of Stress, Anxiety, and Depression.........45
1.15 Examining Whether You Are in Control................................48
1.16 Examining Your Power to Project Yourself Positively 49
1.17 Key Points to Remember 49

CHAPTER TWO: THE GOAL AND A PLAN OF ACTION TO STOP SMOKING..**51**
2.1 Introduction...51
2.2 How to Formulate the Goal to Stop Smoking Now!......................51
2.3 How to Define Your Goal...55
2.4 Key Point to Remember...61
2.5 Problem: The 60 Cigarettes a Day Smoker.................................61
2.6 Stop Smoking Now! Goal: To Stop Smoking NOW!......................62
2.7 How to Make an Action Plan for the Goal: To Stop Smoking NOW!...64
2.8 Action Plan 1: Expressing Self Belief.......................................64
2.9 Action Plan 2: Act with Positive belief and, Show this in Attitudes about Smoking..64
2.10 Action Plan 3: Translating Action 2 into Positive Practical Action..65
2.11 Action Plan 4: Be Confident in the Knowledge that You Are now a non-smoker...65
2.12 Action Plan 5: Affirm the Goal...66
2.13 How to Acquire the Will to Succeed in Giving up Smoking.......67

CHAPTER THREE: STOP SMOKING COMPLETELY, EASILY, AND EFFECTIVELY...**71**
3.1 Deep Relaxation as Weapon to Stop Smoking.............................71
3.2 Practice Sessions..72
3.3 The Dynamics of Mental Prompts...76
3.4 Exercises to Stop Smoking..80
3.5 Positive Suggestions to Stop Smoking......................................96
3.6 How to make the habit of Non-smoking Your Reality..................99
3.7 Going for Your Success to Stop Smoking with Confidence........100
3.8 Practice Sessions..101
3.9 Affirmations to Bring the Results that You Desire......................104

CHAPTER FOUR: RECAPITULATION OF SOME ESSENTIAL POINTS 109

4.1 The Logic of Numbers 109

4.2 The Magic of Success 110

4.3 The Pitfalls of Negative Prompts 110

4.4 Action is the Route to Change 111

4.5 Belief is the Ultimate 111

REFERENCES..115

INTRODUCTION

It is all in the state of mind, success in anything you do begins in the mind.

I.1 The Basic Idea of the Mind Technique in This Book

This book is a practical application of some of the ideas and fundamental principles of mind power techniques which I use in my work and in the regular public workshops that I organise. Some of the workshops have been on memory techniques to enable remembering, techniques to lose weight and techniques to stop smoking.

The book reveals the secret power of the mind and gives the individual the power to achieve success by making use of those secrets. The book presents a novel approach to stop smoking which is simple, fun to practise and highly effective. It demonstrates a unique practical mind technique that enables the individual to stop smoking easily, completely, effectively and effortlessly.

The book contains some of the essential secret weapons which an individual requires, to look good and feel good in every way and regain the energy and stamina that he or she has lost by the ravages of tar and nicotine from inhaling tobacco smoke into the lungs in smoking cigarettes, cigars or pipe. The book teaches a special method of relaxation that enables the individual wishing to stop smoking to accomplish his or her objectives quickly and effectively.

In practising the special method of deep relaxation which I introduce the book, some people may feel light and weightless when they relax. They may feel as light as if they can just float away. It is usual to feel this way but it is not a necessary part of the application of this method. What is necessary is that the individual must feel relaxed.

However, if an individual can feel light during the moment of deep relaxation, he or she is beginning to acquire the feeling of being in control. This is the feeling which this book creates for individuals as they inculcate the habit of relaxation in the special way that I teach it in this book.

When a person has the feeling of being in control constantly in his or her mind, he or she will know that he or she is beginning to accomplish the goal to stop smoking. This is because success in anything that one does begins in the mind. The next stage is for the individual to translate the feeling into the physical activities that will make the feeling become his or her reality so that he or she can experience the real action of giving up smoking and do so easily and effortlessly.

The simple mind techniques in this book are intended to enable any individual to harness the power to bring about the changes which he or she requires in life. These techniques are easily applicable in whatever he or she is doing, whether it is in giving up smoking or in any other venture where the goal of the individual is to achieve success.

This book shows the way to achieve success in giving up smoking and it shows, truly, the way to achieve success in any goal or anything you do; how to be what you want to be, how to do things seriously in a positive way so that you do them successfully. It shows how to erect a solid foundation to the mind castles which people build from day to day.

The strong message in the book is that you will get what you want for what you want is what you get. This means that when you have a positive mental attitude and your mind is fully focused on what you want, the goals which you aspire to attain become easily attainable by you.

Any person who has a sincere desire to stop smoking would be successful with the programme to stop smoking. The person will do so easily and effectively if he or she has a positive mental attitude and a strong belief in his or her own ability to attain the desired objective. The person will stop smoking easily and effectively.

The success comes through an intentional positive action. Any person who can talk the talk about a desire to stop smoking must put the talk into practical action and walk the walk to realize the goal. This book is about responsible positive action which brings about positive changes by helping the individual to stop smoking easily and effectively.

This book shows you how to inculcate a positive mental attitude, how to esteem yourself, how to acquire belief in yourself and eliminate the negativism of doubt, how to project a positive self image in whatever you do. The book takes you through the actions that you must perform, and the attitudes that you must adopt to achieve your goal and stop smoking successfully.

If you believe that you have the power within you to bring to reality anything that you can conceive as possible in your life, then you will be truly successful in achieving your desired objective. You will stop smoking and you will do so easily and effortlessly. Your belief that you will be successful in what you are about to do is a vital requisite for the achievement of your success in the particular goal that you wish to accomplish.

The conception of the idea of positive possibility of success in what you are about to do, and the reality of it, begin with effective thought bricks which form the foundation of your own mind castle in relation to stop smoking easily, effectively and effortlessly. This idea will become much clearer to you in chapter one when I describe the fundamental principles of the mind technique that I introduce to you in this book.

The claim of this book is that every individual has the power within him or her to achieve the goals and objectives that he or she wishes to achieve in life, to make whatever changes he or she wishes to make in his or her life successfully. To do this seriously and conscientiously, the individual must do two very essential things that will bring about the required success as follows.

The first is that the individual must acknowledge the enormous power within him or her. Secondly, the individual must make use of that power by doing something new or, at least, doing something different from what he or she has been doing in the past.

The emphasis here, as in 'walk the walk', mentioned above, is in the positive action which consists in the practise of the relaxation exercises in this book, doing something new or different, to accomplish one's goals and aspirations.

A person's acknowledgement and utilization of his or her inner power for success entails the belief that there is no limit to what he or she can accomplish, legitimately, with his or her mind except the limitations which he or she, wilfully, imposes on himself or herself by distorted thoughts, negative thoughts, and self-doubt. The power of the mind is utilized in thought processes and this is manifested by an individual's actions in so far as thoughts precede actions.

By following all the positive ideas in this book and the actions that they invoke, the serious reader will develop a positive attitude towards the desired goal to stop smoking. This will help him or her to stop smoking easily and effectively.

The reader will also develop a great confidence in his or her ability to succeed in any chosen venture and he or she will be ready, willing, and able to embark on the road to success. The essential ingredients that are required for a recipe for success in the goal to stop smoking by the method of deep relaxation and psychodynamics programming are in this book.

The effective use of these essential ingredients will propel any serious reader to the road of success in the goal to stop smoking. The individual will stop smoking easily and effortlessly when he or she has read the book attentively from the beginning to the end and practised the techniques of relaxation as advised in this book.

A person's decision to read this book brings that person a step nearer to that road; and he or she will be walking firmly on that road with the head held high by the time he or she has read to the end of this book when he or she has read the book with concentrated attention supported by a clear understanding and performance of the necessary actions which an individual must take to achieve the success that he or she desires. Some of these actions consist in practising all the relaxation exercises for giving up smoking which are given in this book.

There is a clear user-friendly advantage to this book which is in the way that things look familiar to the reader as he or she reads through the pages of the book. This is partly because of the simplicity of the ideas that I introduce in this book, the relaxation exercises and the way in which the ideas have been presented in this book, and partly because the subject matter, '*Stop Smoking*', is a subject which is of great public interest. Many people have an interest to stop smoking but they deter themselves from the attempt to stop smoking, with pathetic excuses.

This book provokes the reader into positive action. It urges the reader to avoid the temptation of using pathetic excuses to hold on to an unwanted, unhealthy and dangerous habit. It urges him or her to do something as a positive concern for his or her health, to practise the simple techniques discussed in the book because simple techniques always work. They work because they are simple.

In my work as a psychodynamics analyst and lecturer in London, I organize regular seminars and workshops on psychodynamics techniques such as memory techniques to enable remembering with reference to examination candidates, techniques to lose weight, and the many techniques which I give here to enable you to stop smoking. The seminars and workshops are held regularly at various venues in London, and have been very successful. I have also worked on the subject of sports translating the principles of psychodynamics into the practical areas of sports performance.

In this respect, I have used some of the simple psychodynamics techniques discussed in this book to help my clients, many sports people, athletes, boxers, footballers, gymnasts, and tennis players, to lose weight, stop smoking and to gain a great confidence in themselves. My work with these sports people has enabled them to achieve success in their own sports by attaining a much desired, personal best (PB) performance in their sports.

In view of the great successes of my sports clients, I have every confidence in anyone reading this book with the serious purpose to stop smoking. If this is your intention for reading this book, you must spend time to try out all the positive suggestions given and participate fully in the deep relaxation exercises given in *the practice sessions* in the book.

I.2 The Practice Sessions

There are many exercises in this book because it is a practical book to stop smoking. I show you how to perform the exercises. You must perform them in order to stop smoking. As I mentioned above, if a person can talk the talk about stop smoking, then that person must be prepared to put the talk into practical action and walk the walk which will lead him or her to the fulfilment of the desired goal. The *practice sessions* are an essential part of the positive action in this book and they are intended to help the serious reader to develop a relaxed attitude in mind and body. This will help him or her to focus the mind sharply on the desired objective to stop smoking.

I.3 The Key Points to Remember

The *key points to remember* which are given in the various sections of this book are a quick reference to the issues raised in a preceding discussion and provide a quick summary of the key points in the discussion. The act of remembering these key points forms part of the practical action in this book for it is important to remember the ideas so that one can put them into practice.

This book is an exploration into the powers of the human mind. My underlying thesis is that success in anything that a person does begins in the mind. *It is all in the mind.* This becomes obvious as one reads through the pages of this book. As I mentioned above, if you are reading this book with a serious intention to stop smoking, you must practise the simple techniques in the book because simple techniques work. They work because they are simple. The simple techniques in this book are part of the simple techniques that I use every week in my own work and in the workshops that I have mentioned above.

I.4 Further Useful Secret Programmes in the Book

In addition to helping readers to learn how to stop smoking completely, easily and effectively, the readers will also learn the following secrets from reading the book.

- ❖ The secrets of how the mind works.
- ❖ How to use effective thought bricks to erect an impregnable mind castle.
- ❖ How to relax and take control of any situation.
- ❖ How to recognise the effects of stress and anxiety in personal life.
- ❖ How to acquire confidence, self esteem and self worth.
- ❖ How to formulate goals and plan for their achievement.
- ❖ How to draw out an action plan to achieve a specific goal.
- ❖ How to visualise for success in any venture.

I.5 Exude Confidence Always

Always be confident in what you do and in yourself as a human being. This book teaches you some mind techniques which will help you to stop smoking. If you are reading the book with the specific intention to stop smoking, you must be confident and persistent so that you will be successful and, stop smoking, easily and effectively.

To doubt yourself and your own ability to cope from the start is negative. To understand this, you must know that doubt is a thought brick and negative thought bricks lead, disastrously, to failure.

An anxiety can bring about a negative thought brick. Here is an illustration of how dysthymic anxiety can lead to doubt via the defence mechanism of rationalisation. Some hardened smokers challenged me at one of my *Stop Smoking* workshops. They asked me: how can you write a book about stop smoking when you have never been a smoker?

My answer is simple. This book is not about how to be a smoker. This book is about how to stop smoking. It is about being a non-smoker, like me. In this book, I am teaching you how to be what I am, a non-smoker. It is a book that raises awareness to some of the destructive health problems that smokers might have and the book guides smokers through the process of the cessation of smoking.

Also, I can write a book about *Stop Smoking* because I have all the credentials to write such book. I am a health professional, I am a non-smoker and, as I mentioned above, I have run regular workshops for smoking cessation for many years.

You might, also, like to know that I have used some of the techniques that I introduce to you here, to help cancer patients who are hospitalized and, also, to help some pregnant women to give birth painlessly without epidural. None of these patients asked me how can you help a cancer patient when you have never had cancer? Or, how can you help a pregnant woman to give birth painlessly when you have never given birth to a child or ever been pregnant?

These questions manifest the questioners' anxieties. They are already planning an excuse for failure before the attempt. Do you think that all the midwives and nurses in a maternity hospital have been pregnant and given birth to babies? Remember that some of them are men. Alternatively, do you think that all the people involved in the treatment of cancer patients in a cancer hospital have all had cancer?

What has happened with the hardened smokers is that with them, the anxiety of smoking has become dysthymic and led them to the negative route of doubt through the defence mechanism of rationalisation. They doubt their own ability to succeed, but they rationalize their doubt as in a doubt of a book which they have never seen or read. This is their anxiety giving rise to lack of confidence. It appeases the wish to avoid the burden of reading the book, and sustains their smoker status.

Thus, in this way, the attempt to stop smoking ends up in smoke in an abject failure. Remember that if you focus on doubt, this will be retained in the unconscious and failure will become your reality. This is because doubt is your dominant thought brick. You will understand this better in the pages of this book. Refer to *thought bricks* in section 1.2 below.

I have mentioned how smoking can be due to dysthymic anxiety which comes through the negative route of doubt by rationalization above. In this way the individual always defends his or her smoking action. I shall give further explanation to the defence mechanism, *rationalization,* which is employed in anxiety problems as in my explanation above with the defence of the doubters.

I.6 The Idea of Psycho-cybernetics

However, you can also view this book as an introduction to psycho-cybernetics, the application of solid thought bricks as a foundation for the construction of mind castles in making radical changes in life. In this respect, the book is a journey into a new world, a new way of doing things, a new method of approach to personal and social problems, a journey into oneself, a quest for the development of the self.

I shall take you on the journey or quest in the next chapter with a preparatory exercise to set the psychical system in motion so that you will feel relaxed. When you perform this exercise properly, diligently, you will notice that you will feel relaxed in mind and body from that moment onwards.

CHAPTER ONE: ESSENTIAL PRELIMINARY STEPS TO STOP SMOKING

When you visualize something, you can make it a material reality. If you can visualize yourself as a non-smoker and think constantly that you are a non-smoker, then this will certainly become your reality. This is the power of visualization: whatever you visualize, you can realize it.

This book sets out to show you how to bring about the reality by the effective use of the powers of your mind. It takes you on a journey into a new world of infinite positive possibilities where all wishes are granted. Your wish to stop smoking will be granted to you here because you are serious about it.

1.1 The Preparatory Exercise

Now let us begin our quest for success in giving up smoking with a preparatory exercise which takes us to a new world of positive possibilities. The purpose of this is twofold. First, it prepares an individual for the regime of positive thinking and deep relaxation of mind and body through diaphragmatic breathing. Secondly, it underlines the role of visualisation in mental activities. The preparatory exercise will enable you to feel relaxed constantly.

It is important to feel relaxed and be relaxed most of the time because with relaxation an individual can do things easily and effectively. With relaxation, your goal to stop smoking will be accomplished easily and effortlessly. In this way, the habit of relaxation will become your everyday reality. In this exercise, I shall take you to a world of positive possibilities where all wishes are granted, all goals and desires accomplished and all dreams fulfilled. It is, indeed, a world of positive thinking which empowers you and enables you to eliminate self-doubt.

Sit down comfortably on a chair or couch and let us start on our journey. Breathe in through your diaphragm. Hold your breath for a mental count from five to zero. Five, four, three, two, one, z e r o. (Try to count out the *z e r o*....as you breathe out, and feel the effect).

Now, gently breathe out slowly and go deeper, deeper, deeper and deeper into relaxation. You will feel relaxed immediately but if you do not feel relaxed, continue the breathing exercise until you feel relaxed.

As you are now relaxed, I want you to empty your mind of all doubts, all negative thoughts and mental distortions. Now, I want you to go deeper and deeper into relaxation so that with each breath that you take and at each moment your sense and feeling of relaxation will increase within your mind and body. I want you to learn that from this moment onwards the word **R E L A X** *will bring instant deep relaxation to your mind and body so that whatever situation you are in, wherever you are, you will be absolutely relaxed and in total control, come what may.*

Now, I want you to imagine that you are listening to the sound of my voice or, the sound of your own voice if you have recorded the instructions that I give to you here on a media tool for your own convenience. Now as I (or you) count the numbers, slowly, down from 10 to zero, you will go ten times more deeply relaxed and you will be relaxed on each, and every descending number. Every number down will be a step to peace, tranquillity and total deep relaxation for you. The number now is ten, nine, eight, seven, six, five, four, three, two, one, you are now drifting, shifting, going deeper, deeper, deeper, all the way to z e r o.

You are now very, very, very deeply relaxed. I want you to know that some people feel a tingling sensation when they are relaxed by this method, others have a feeling of elation, some others feel very light and weightless, as light and weightless as if they can float away. A few other people feel heavy as they are laden with negative thoughts. At this moment, whatever positive feeling you have is right and proper for you. So, stay with your positive feeling as you go deeper, deeper and deeper into relaxation.

Now I want you to come with me for a journey to a new world. This is the world of positive possibilities. It is a world of goodness, a world where you can do good deeds and achieve your goals. You can achieve beneficial results and obtain whatever you want in the world of positive possibilities without harming or undermining anyone. It is a world in which you eliminate negative thoughts and self-doubts from your life.

In this world, you can get whatever positive thing you want because whatever positive thing you want is what you get. Every positive wish is granted in this world. Your wish to stop smoking is a positive wish which will be granted in the world of positive possibilities. There is an abundance of good wishes and beneficial things for everyone in this world.

In this world of positive possibilities, all your wishes and desires are fulfilled. You can stop smoking easily, completely, effectively and effortlessly in this world. Now, before we can go to the world of positive possibilities, I want you to become aware of some of the critical health and social reasons to stop smoking which make this journey to the world of positive possibilities a necessary journey. I want you to deliberate on those reasons for a moment before you make the journey.

- ❖ *Smoking is poisonous. It poisons and destroys your lungs with tar and nicotine.*
- ❖ *Smoking affects the immune system and makes the smoker more vulnerable to illnesses and diseases.*
- ❖ *Smoking affects the smoker's sex life. It lowers the female's fertility rate and reduces sperm count in men.*
- ❖ *Smoking leads to the threat of bronchitis and emphysema.*
- ❖ *Smoking causes bad breath, bad cough, irritability, nervousness and tension.*
- ❖ *Smoking saps a person's energy, strength and stamina making it difficult for the person to take part in active competitive sports.*
- ❖ *Smoking is a very old fashioned, unhealthy, and unhygienic habit and it is now forbidden on aeroplane journeys and many public places.*
- ❖ *Smoking is now an anti-social habit.*
- ❖ *Smoking is a form of self punishment from perverted pleasure in a Sado-Masochistic sort of way since smokers knowingly inflict*

damage on themselves by smoking in opposition to public health warning about the dangers of smoking.

- ❖ *Smokers are callous. They have no conscience about forcing other people and children around them to become unwilling passive smokers to their own detriment.*
- ❖ *The Hollywood image of smokers is now very old-hat. The idea which it conjures in the minds of smokers is unhealthy and it has lived past its sell by date and use by date. We are now in a new age, a new millennium of health care and health consciousness.*

In respect of these health and social reasons and many other personal reasons to stop smoking, you have chosen to go to the world of positive possibilities to stop smoking completely, easily and effectively.

Now, I want you to visualize yourself in the world of positive possibilities. Be there at the count of three to zero. The number now is three, two, one, zero.

You are now in the new world of positive possibilities. You can climb the highest mountain, bungee jump, parachute jump down from the greatest height. You can, accomplish a seemingly impossible feat in the world of positive possibilities. Everything that is positive is possible in this world. Every good wish and positive goal that you want to achieve is easily achievable in this world.

Whatever goal you accomplish in the world of positive possibilities will also be accomplished and retained by you in the real world. Here are powerful words of assurance given from the source of inner energy force to assure you, energize you, and guarantee the certainly of your success as follows.

"So, I say to you, Ask and it will be given to you; search, and you will find; knock, and the door will be opened for you. For everyone who asks receives, and everyone who searches finds, and for everyone who knocks, the door will be opened." (Luke 11, 9-10).

It is the same for you here in the world of positive possibilities. Your positive wishes will be granted here for that is why you are here. So, use your time here wisely and beneficially, profitably, because what you wish for, what you asked for, will be yours.

Now I want you to visualize yourself as a non-smoker. I want you to stay with the knowledge that in this world, you will accomplish your goal easily and effortlessly.

Your positive belief, your optimism and the positive energy which you invest on your positive thoughts, and your desire to stop smoking will help you to accomplish your wishes. Now I want you to accomplish your goal to stop smoking completely in the time that you have in the new world of positive possibilities.

This is your moment, *the moment of positive action and positive accomplishment, the moment of healthy living for you. You know what you need to do to eliminate smoking from your life completely. Do it now in this opportune moment.*

As you are now busy with the accomplishment of your goal to stop smoking easily, completely, effectively and effortlessly, I will leave you for a moment for you to complete what you are doing and become a non-smoker easily and effectively. You will be successful in what you are doing and you will accomplish every positive wish or desire that you need to accomplish because every positive wish is granted in the world of positive possibilities and will be retained by you in the real world, they will be actualized by you in the world of actuality.

Be empowered and energised by the powerful words of assurance coming from the source of inner energy force to assure you and guarantee your success.

I will leave you now for you to accomplish your goal. By the time that I return, you will become a non-smoker. You will be very deeply relaxed and absolutely in control, and this is how things will be with you from this moment onwards. Go on, do what you need to do to accomplish your wish or desire and I will be with you in a moment.

(I will Pause here for you to perform the exercise)

You are deeply relaxed. You feel peaceful and in control. You have done what you need to do, and you have accomplished your goal to stop smoking and you have done so easily and effortlessly. You are now a non-smoker. Every other positive desire that you have is easily achievable by you from now onwards. Believe it for it is true.

At the count of one to five, you will return to the world of actuality where you will actualize your goal to stop smoking and every other positive desire that you may have so that they become real and permanent accomplishments for you. You will be very deeply relaxed, confident, positive, very optimistic and in control.

These feelings will stay with you and be part of your everyday feelings from this moment onwards. The number now is one, two, three, four, five. The number five has been counted. You are welcome to the actual world where you can now actualize your wishes and desires.

NOTE:
You may count the number down to go into relaxation, the higher the number from which you begin your count, the deeper you will relax as follows.

At the count of ten to zero you be very deeply relaxed. The number now is ten, nine, eight, seven, six, five, four, three, two, one, zero. You are now very deeply relaxed.

Count the numbers upwards to come up, sit up and to open your eyes if they were shut. In general, you may count the numbers up or down to perform a specific action in accordance with a specific instruction as follows.

At the count of one to five you will be jumping for joy in the knowledge that you are now a non-smoker. The number now is one, two, three, four, five. You are now a non-smoker.

Where it is necessary to be deeply relaxed and focused to perform a specific action, you may count down as follows.

At the count of five to zero you will be deeply relaxed, and you will be inside your body to clean out your lungs. Five, four, three, two, one, zero. You are now inside your body. Your job now is to clean out your lungs. (Refer to chapter 3.4 for the full details of this powerful exercise).

Now, if you have performed the above preparatory exercise diligently and successfully, the other exercises in this book will become great fun for you because the preparatory exercise sets the pattern of the fun activities in this book.

As I stated above, the preparatory exercise has a dual purpose. First, it prepares an individual for the regime of positive thinking and deep relaxation in mind and body through diaphragmatic breathing. Secondly, it underlines the role of visualization in mental activities. If you can visualize it, you can realize it, that is, make it real.

If you can visualize yourself as a non-smoker in the world of positive possibilities, you will be able to stop smoking easily, completely and effortlessly in the actual world of here and now.

Visualization is a mental process by which an individual uses positive rational thought to create mental pictures of his or her goals, wishes or desires. It is called *Creative Visualisation* because of its enormous creative potential. The mental pictures help the individual to turn goals, wishes or desires into reality. In short, visualization is the act of the construction of mind castles.

If you can bring thought and picture together about you giving up smoking and seeing yourself in the picture as a non-smoker, you are conceiving a potent idea, building up something tangible, constructing mind castles. Any wishes, desires, intentions or major goals which you can conceive in this way, is easily achievable by you. What you need next is the patience and the right frame of mind to put a rock, solid foundation to the castles which you have built in your mind.

However, you can also accomplish your goals, wishes and desire even if you lack the power of visualisation or the ability to form mental images of what you want. It is sufficient to have an idea of what you want to accomplish and then bring it about through other means which are discussed in this book. A sound knowledge of the fundamental principles discussed here will help you immensely to accomplish any goal or desire.

1.2 The Fundamental Principles of the Mind Technique

Now I want you to come with me to begin your quest for success in your goal to stop smoking right away by examining the fundamental principles of the mind power techniques that I introduce in this book. These principles are the rock, solid foundation to your mind castles and a constant adherence to them will help you to understand what is involved in the use of the power of the mind to make positive changes in your life.

A constant adherence to these principles will enable you to accomplish your goals, wishes and desires. If you understand these principles and act on them constantly, then you will find that giving up smoking will be fun and easy for you.

In general, you will get what you want for what you want is what you get. The mind techniques which I present throughout this book are based on the general operation of the human mind in relation to a certain belief of the individual. Thus, to understand and master the practical mind techniques for giving up smoking easily and effectively, it is essential that the individual understands the cardinal principles in the mind techniques and apply them generally in one's actions. When this happens constantly the principles will become part of the routine of everyday motor behaviour for the individual.

1. The Thought Bricks of the Mind

Thoughts are the building blocks of both mental and physical constructions. The thought bricks of the mind can either enhance an individual's power to give up smoking or they can restrict the individual's effort to give up smoking. Thoughts are in the mind and they are the bricks with which we build our impregnable mind castles.

In order to build castles in the air or on land, one needs solid and effective thought bricks to lay the foundation of the castle. This principle of mind power stipulates that whatever thoughts you repeat powerfully and often enough will become realities for you. For example, if you are thinking positive thoughts about giving up smoking such as, *I will give up smoking easily and effectively* this will become your reality if the thoughts are powerful and constant in your mind.

The thoughts, whatever they are, which you have in your mind the most often will materialise into reality for you. As in the example above, if you affirm or repeat your thoughts of success in giving up smoking, you will achieve success in giving up smoking steadily, easily and effectively. As mentioned above, if you are thinking positive thoughts about your success in giving up smoking this will become your reality. This applies to any goals, wishes or desires that you may have.

On the other hand, if you are preoccupied with self doubts and negative thoughts about what you want to do, constantly thinking about failures and difficulties, failure and difficulties will become your reality.

The general rule for the application of this principle is to have a positive mental attitude and think positive thoughts so that positive feelings will flow to you, automatically, which will lead you to the achievement of positive results in your life. Thoughts are the bricks of all building structures. Thoughts are in the mind. If your thoughts are all about success you will be successful, if you think mostly about failure, this will become your reality!

If you are always doubting yourself and doubting everything, you must remember that 'doubt' is a thought brick. If 'doubt' is the thought that you have most often in your mind, your 'doubt' will become your reality. Your doubt erases your positive thought and gives you the realisation of failure. If you doubt your ability to give up smoking, if your doubt is the thought that you have most often in your mind, you will prove yourself right by your doubt and fail to give up smoking.

You will get what you think about for what you think about is what you get. You will give up smoking easily and effectively if you think that you will give up smoking, easily and effectively and believe from now onwards that you will give up smoking easily and effectively. This is the reason why you are reading this book. You must justify your reason by a positive belief in your reason and in yourself.

Your belief in the idea of success is a positive thought that stirs your mind to positive efforts and leads you to success. Negative thoughts and self doubts dampen the edge of positive action because they stir your mind away from your chosen objective and thus, lead you to failure and disappointment.

This first fundamental principle of the operation of the mind is vital in everything that we do, the plans and the decisions that we make from day to day. The operation of this first principle is embodied in the functions of the unconscious mind which I shall discuss below in this chapter.

If what you want to do is not quite clear in your mind, one way to tackle it is to see the problem as a challenge which must be confronted. In this way, you will be inspired to investigate the solution and find out more about it.

If your reaction to a problem is negative and you adopt a negative attitude just to avoid the problem or, if you run away completely from the problem, you may find that you will be running away each time you perceive something as a problem.

You will not solve any problem by running away from it. Thus, if the supposed problem concerns your goals and aspirations, then you will find that the goals will not be achieved by running away from them.

2. There is a Limitless Intrinsic Power within Everyone
The power of the human mind is awesome. It can bring great results when it is used in a positive way and it can cause a lot of problems, disaster and ruin when used in a negative way.

I want you to understand that the power of your mind is potentially unlimited, that is, you have an unlimited potential within you now to accomplish anything you wish and an unlimited potential within you to achieve positive results in your life, including the power to give up smoking even now, easily and effectively. Believe it for it is true.

There is no limit to the power of your mind except those limitations which you wilfully impose on your mind by yourself through negative thoughts. The power of the human mind is ingenious and prodigious. This ingenuity of the human mind enables humans to design sophisticated computers but, the power of your mind is much greater than that of the most sophisticated computer because the computer is designed by human mind and it is, by itself, unoriginal.

The power of your mind is there with you throughout your life from the moment of your birth. You can control your entire life with your mind. The magic of success in anything you do is within you. It is within your mind. Your mind is the magic power through which you achieve great success in whatever you do.

The essence of this second principle is that acknowledging the prodigious power of your mind will help you to give up smoking now, easily and effectively, because you know that you have the power within you to give up smoking now. With your constant practise of increased deep relaxation, the simple psychodynamics programmes in this book are easily assimilated in your mind as you read this book.

3. The Principle of Universal Energy

There is a universal energy within everyone. You can channel this energy to your desired goals and aspirations by way of your attitudes. As in the points that I made above, positive attitudes toward your goals channel positive energy and negative attitudes and self doubts channel negative energy which leads to lack of fulfilment or disappointment.

Personal energies help to determine the success or failure of your goals and aspirations. The energy which you channel into what you do and, in the opposite, the energy which you attract, both determine how your attitude towards your major goals, your immediate objectives and your life in general relates to what you desire to create for yourself. These energies also relate to the extent, or urgency of your desire.

The essential question for you here is how to determine what may need to change or evolve within you in order to transform you into a powerfully attractive force of energy so you can bring your goal, objectives, or dreams such as 'stop smoking now!' into reality. You can manifest your goals and desires more effectively by channelling positive attitudes towards them with greater expectation of their realization. In other words, the energy of your belief helps to make reality of your goals. Refer also to the first principle above.

In our everyday motor activities, each one of us channels his or her energy as dictated by his or her attitudes, feelings and beliefs to obtain the results he or she requires. Although occasionally, unfortunately, it happens that the energy of the individual is channelled negatively, and the individual obtains the result that he or she does not require.

The universal energy which is in everyone can also be manifested in a different way in every action of the individual because the individual attracts energy and also radiates energy into the universe by his or her attitudes towards events and situations in his or her life. The energy is manifest in the life of individuals by the state of affairs in their lives such as abundant wealth and prosperity, happiness, success in any venture, destitution, romantic bliss, confidence, positive feeling, negative feeling and many others.

Also, as in the above examples, other ways in which the energy can be manifested in an individual's life are in being rich and prosperous, being romantically happy, feeling rejected and alone, feeling inferior, feeling unworthy for success and so forth. All the ways to manifest the energy are within you because the energy is in you. The energy can manifest success, happiness, abundant wealth and prosperity much easier than it can manifest failure and destitution because the natural state of the universe is for happiness, wealth, prosperity and abundance.

There is also a central dynamic pure energy force of magnetic power of creativity which is within everyone. The knowledge of this inner magnetic power within you should enable you to change the pattern of your thought and belief system and make them beneficial for you. You can do great things and achieve great goals if you believe that you have a dynamic, pure energy force of magnetic power within you to attract the things you wish in life by your attitudes and your actions.

This is an essential doctrine in depth psychology and it entails the belief that if you think that you can do it, you can. If you believe that you can stop smoking now, then so be it, you can. The force and energy of your belief engenders positive action to realize your wish. This book teaches you to believe that you can, and to always believe that you can, in everything that you do in the general affairs of your life.

You can see quite clearly from what I have been saying here about energy, that success in anything, success in giving up smoking easily and effectively is within you. Success in giving up smoking easily and effectively is a universal energy which is an integral part of the natural limitless, intrinsic latent power which is within you.

Refer to the second principle above. Success and wealth are external expression of abundance but the energy of abundance which causes the success and wealth to manifest in your life is internal. Thus, you can see from this that the magic of success is truly within you. Your success in giving up smoking now is within you because you have the power now to take positive actions to eliminate smoking from your life.

4. Every Individual is the Architect of his own Life
Every, adult, individual is responsible for the state of affairs of his or her own life. As a result of an individual's thought patterns in general he or she is responsible for the way and manner he or she makes progress or failure on this planet in respect of the choices and decisions that he or she makes according to how and where his or her thoughts lead to in the execution of a particular action. It is not right for an individual to defend himself or herself for his or her failures and lack of progress at any venture by blaming the state, other people, or by blaming God in appealing to the arguments for determinism, predestination, or fatalism.

You have the freedom to change your life by changing the pattern of your thoughts in making them more positive and beneficial to you. This is an essential principle of the power of the mind. You are the architect of your life and you can change your life by changing the pattern of your thoughts.

To profit from this principle, you must proceed by seeking for ways in which you can take complete control of your life, develop your ideas by making them more positive and beneficial to you, become more and more assertive and self-reliant, and less and less dependent on other people for assistance.

5. Action is a positive expression of thought.
The principle of positive action which I have mentioned above is an essential ingredient in a recipe for success in any goal. If it matters to you then the onus is on you to do something about it. If you are truly convinced that you need to give up smoking then you must act positively to stop smoking now!

In your actions, you must always act with conviction. If you are giving a positive message to yourself or reading out your own affirmations, you must always act with the conviction that your message is going to be received by your unconscious mind and that your wishes and intentions will be realised, that is, made real.

The essential maxim for action which you must always remember here is that *everything that you believe to be true is true or becomes true for you.* Remember what I said above under the second principle that if you think you can, you can. If you believe that you can do it, you can. No one is ready for success in any venture unless he or she believes that he or she can achieve it.

This is an incontrovertible thesis of the power of the mind. Always endeavour to be enthusiastic in what you do and act with absolute faith in your expectation of success. This part about your expectation is also included in your manifestation of the energy to bring about the desired result.

Remember that we are dealing here with positive action which is provoked by positive thoughts and, always avoid the temptation to follow the negative pattern of finger pointing, that is, blaming other people such as, for example, your partner, the government, tobacco companies, cigarette manufacturers or the supermarkets when things go wrong in your attempt to give up smoking. Take responsibility for your own affairs and do something about it by taking positive action to effect desired changes in your life.

With respect to our first principle which is a cardinal thesis of the power of the mind, it is important to realise that the power of thought is the essence of the mind. The influential French philosopher, Rene Descartes (1596-1650) saw this during his great meditations which led him to assert his famous maxim, *Cogito Ergo Sum* (I think therefore, I am) in his writings, *Discourse on Method* (1637) and *Meditations on First Philosophy* (1641). Descartes saw *thinking* as the indubitable proof of man's existence.

Descartes was very well aware of the great powers of the mind because most of his influential ideas in his books came from his series of dreams, the *Olympica* dreams of 10 November, 1619. These dreams enabled the development of his vortex theory of science.

The operation of thinking is a function of the mind. The thinking power of the mind is clearly illustrated in all the deliberations and cogitations which Descartes went through in his meditations and all his other ruminative activities to establish the certainty of the *Cogito*. Descartes could have equally said, *Credo Ergo Sum* (I believe therefore, I am) as your belief is important in arriving at the result you require. Remember that belief is also a thought brick. Refer to the first principle above.

For you to acquire the technique of mind power and to build effective mind castles, you must always be able to apply the above fundamental principles of mind power generally in everything you do in your everyday life with respect to your thinking patterns with regard to whatever projects or goals you have. For the purpose in this book, the project or goal is giving up smoking. The fundamental principles mentioned above are applied in the techniques which I discuss in this book together with the secret of how the human mind works.

1.3 Key Points to Remember

- ❖ Your thoughts are the bricks for mental constructions. Positive thoughts give solid foundation to your building projects and help you to give up smoking easily and effortlessly. Negative thoughts dampen the edge of positive action, lead to failure, destruction, disappointment, and ruin.

- ❖ The power of your mind is limitless. Acknowledging this power enables you to know that you can achieve whatever you put your mind to. Thus, the magic of success in giving up smoking is truly within you, it is in your positive acknowledgement of the principles we have discussed above in relation to your thoughts about giving up smoking.

- ❖ There is a universal energy within you, which manifests success or failure according to your thought patterns in relation to your goal of giving up smoking.

- ❖ You are the architect of your own life. You have the power to effect changes in your life because it is up to you and not other people.

- ❖ Acknowledge that you have the power of a dynamic creative energy force within you which, when recognised, enables you to bring about positive changes in your life.

- ❖ The power of your mind is greater than that of the most sophisticated computer because the computer is created by the ingenuity of the human mind.

- ❖ Remember that action speaks louder than words and act positively to bring about the changes which you seek.

1.4 The Secrets of How the Mind Works

We can learn a great deal about how the mind works by examining the levels of mental awareness, or the levels of consciousness, if you like. The advantage of this is that by knowing how the mind functions you will be in a better position to direct your thoughts to greater, more positive, and beneficial, purposes and achieve the results that you desire. This will help you to programme your mind more effectively with appropriate mental prompts to help you to give up smoking easily, effectively, and effortlessly.

An individual's knowledge of how the mind works will enable the individual to appreciate the powers of his or her memory as a facet of the mind and then to achieve the result that he or she desires by using his or her memory to his or her own advantage. I am concerned here with the quality of consciousness in psychical topography.

When you read this book with a serious intention to give up smoking you will find, easily and quickly, that the deep relaxation exercises and the positive suggestions in the book will become part of your memory which is, in this respect, your unconscious mind. This is where the ideas need to be, to form part of your motor activity.

The human mind functions at three principal levels. These levels have been clearly recognised within the field of depth psychology, that is, the psychology of the dynamic forces in the interaction between conscious and unconscious mental processes. These levels are more appropriately perceived as levels of mental awareness, hence I have described them, jointly, as the quality of consciousness. They are as follows.

The Conscious Level
This is the level of everyday waking life. You are now reading this book at the conscious level of your mental functioning if you are aware that you are reading this book and know fully well that you are reading it and why you are reading it. The conscious level of mental function is the level of operation when one is awake and so at this level one can reason, criticise and control voluntary action. Your decision to give up smoking is made at this level.

The Preconscious Level
This is the level of latent ideas which have the potentiality of becoming conscious at anytime. For instance, there were some things which happened to you last year, last month, yesterday or last week and some other things which you caused to happen last week, yesterday, last month or last year in so far as their occurrence was the direct result of your own action.

As I have now got your undivided attention because you are listening to me, attentively, at this moment in reading this book, your mind is not concentrating on the events of yesterday, last week, last month or last year because it is occupied with the events of the moment in listening to what I am saying to you.

However, since I have now provoked you or stirred up your mind by mentioning the events of yesterday, last week, last month or last year, the flow of thoughts of those events may now come to your mind without difficulty because they have been triggered by my reference to them.

The memories that have now been triggered by my reference to them are said to be at the preconscious level of mental functioning because they are latent memories which are at the threshold of consciousness. They are not being used at any moment, though they are not forgotten.

The Unconscious Level
This level was first investigated by the Viennese neurologist and physiologist, Sigmund Freud (1856-1939), founder of psychoanalysis. He used the term as a way to understand how the mind works and as the basis for the treatment of psychoneurotic disorders. It is the most confused and confusing level of mental functioning.

- ❖ The idea of the inaccessibility of mental items to consciousness due to their repression.
- ❖ The belief that such mental items which are inaccessible are, at the same time, causally active. Unconscious items have the power to affect the individual by giving rise to psychoneurotic symptoms and other puzzling or embarrassing behaviours whose origins have escaped the individual's consciousness because of their repression which makes them inaccessible.
- ❖ The belief that unconscious materials belong to a general psychical system of unconsciousness to which all unconscious materials inhere. This general psychical system is described by Freud as the *system unconscious*.
- ❖ Memories which are stored in the unconscious remain there permanently until released by the individual.

However, for the understanding of the power of the mind, your own unconscious mind is the simple and uncomplicated part of your mental awareness at which your mind is deeply relaxed and is totally uncluttered by bias, criticism, self doubt, tension, general disbelief, etc. At this level the mind faithfully records, reproduces, and controls the entire motor and sensory activities of an individual's life.

In this respect, every experience of an individual's life, every feeling, reaction, emotion, etc. is recorded in the unconscious level of his mind and can be reproduced during moments of deep relaxation. The unconscious is seen, in this sense, as the reservoir of everything that happens in an individual's life and everything that constitutes the individual's personality.

The unconscious can be taken, in this sense, as the totality of an individual's character and attitudes, the storehouse of all memory, and the centre of the individual's habits. I have described this view of the unconscious elsewhere as the *container theory of the mind* (Maurice-Nneke 2003).

In his *Collected Works, Volume 8,* the Swiss psychiatrist, Carl Gustav Jung (1875-1961), founder of the Society of Analytical Psychology and former sidekick of Sigmund Freud, describes the unconscious as a "receptacle of all memories".

With respect to giving up smoking the unconscious level of the mind functions in an automatic way, recording, and reproducing the events of an individual's life. All beliefs, thoughts, feelings, etc, are stored or recorded in the unconscious, the everlasting receptacle and these are reproduced automatically in the individual's thoughts and motor actions.

For example, if a person has negative thoughts and believes that he or she might fail with his or her goal of giving up smoking such belief is stored or recorded in the person's unconscious and reproduced in his or her motor actions. Such a person will not take a positive action to give up smoking because he or she believes that such action will be a failure.

Thus, failure will become his or her reality because he or she thinks about failure. In other words, a person who has a negative attitude towards his or her goal will find that the negative attitude will be recorded in his or her unconscious mind and failure will become his or her reality. Refer to the first fundamental principle discussed above.

On the other hand, if the individual has positive beliefs about himself or herself, his or her goals and aspirations about giving up smoking and feeling fit, healthy, and energetic, these are what will be recorded in the unconscious and they will come true for him or her in his or achievement of positive results in his or her intentions.

The unconscious level controls involuntary action and it is very receptive and active during the state of sleep and in waking state. Remember the first principle of the power of the mind: what you think of most often becomes your reality. This is because what you think of most often is what is recorded in the unconscious mind.

At the unconscious level, all rational thoughts are suspended. Thus, at this level, the mind does not reason, analyse, or criticize. Instead, all thinking processes which are carried out at the conscious level are stored up and played back in the unconscious. Thus, when ideas and beliefs are recorded in the unconscious, whether false or true beliefs, the mind retains them automatically and the ideas, beliefs, thoughts, or feelings are acted out by the individual in motor activity.

This is how your thoughts become your reality. This is how it is possible for you to give up smoking easily and effectively. The positive ideas for giving up smoking that are contained in this book, which I am bringing to you to enable you to give up smoking are the ones which would be retained by your unconscious mind to be acted out in your motor activity!

With respect to this power of the unconscious, you can see clearly from what I have said here that when positive ideas about success in giving up smoking are recorded in the unconscious, the individual automatically thinks positively about achieving success in giving up smoking and in whatever venture he or she engages in.

However, when negative ideas are recorded in the unconscious in relation to the ideas of the subject or venture, the individual shies away from the subject or venture and procrastinates and vacillates about the right things to do or the most appropriate goals to have and ends up with nothing because he or she is unable to decide.

As a matter of information, the term *unconscious*, as used above and throughout this book, has been described in some ancient writings as the *subconscious*. The term subconscious implies an inferior state and does not give an adequate description of the psychodynamics of mental processes.

On the contrary, the unconscious is the most powerful force in the psychodynamics of mental functions. If you wish to know more about the unconscious, refer to my more elaborate book on the subject, (Maurice-Nneke, 2003).

The Supraconscious Level
There is a fourth level of mental awareness known as the *supraconscious* level. This is responsible for direct knowing and it functions independent of ordinary thought processes. It is utilised for extrasensory perception (ESP). ESP is a term which is used to describe four areas of the power of the mind. These are the powers of clairvoyance, precognition, psychokinesis (also known as telekinesis), and telepathy.

Clairvoyance is the power to specifically perceive or know an event or object that is out of the natural range of human knowledge or perception, without the use of ordinarily recognised means of human knowledge or perception. *Precognition* is the power of knowledge of future events in advance of their occurrence without deducing their occurrence from available data. *Psychokinesis* (PK) or *Telekinesis* (TK) is the power to use the mind to cause motion and changes in external objects. *Telepathy,* also known as thought transference, is the power of direct mental communication between two persons who may not necessarily be at close quarters.

A person who is adept in the use of any of these powers of the mind is usually known as a *psychic* and the four areas of the power of the mind mentioned above constitute what is called *psi* (referring to psychic power). However, the term *psi* is also the name of the 23rd letter in the Greek alphabet. This term is usually employed in theories, equations, and experiments to denote an unknown quantity as opposed to what is given or postulated.

Thus, to the world of natural science psi, as denoted by the four areas of the power of the mind given above, is still an unknown quantity despite decades of psychical research by eminent parapsychologists in Britain and the USA. But this is not totally surprising because natural science is slow to absorb new ideas outside its limited boundary and many scientists of the past find the idea of the existence of the mind puzzling or incomprehensible.

Many scientists, as scientists, disdain the idea of the psychical or the mental. They believe that everything is physical. As individuals, however, they may admit to themselves that mind exists otherwise they make no sense when they use the expression 'I have a mind of my own'.

Many people today still scoff at an individual's manifestation of any psi power. For example, the once famous spoon bender, Uri Geller, was well known in the 1970s for his psychokinetic powers yet many people branded him a cheat and a magician at the time of his fame. Even today in the new millennium clairvoyance advertisements are found in the back pages of astrological publications and unpopular magazines.

Some academic people adopt scepticism and cynicism as a mask for their ignorance. Some of these people doubt that the clairvoyants possess any powers of vision and still regard them as charlatans. Some other people wear the 'It's not scientific' (INS) cloak. This is an imaginary cloak of intellectual smugness which confers an illusory sense of superiority to those who wear it while, at the same time, it betrays their lack of knowledge and understanding on a particular topic.

Nothing is very much, more vile and unworthy attitude in academics than intellectual dishonesty which is a pretentious mask of ignorance. Some people find it difficult to give credit to what they are unable to understand or explain scientifically. Thus, they embarrass themselves by seeking refuge in their own limitations of knowledge.

I am not saying that you should endorse the psychics if you have doubts about their claims. Far from it, I believe that if you have genuine doubt, as an educated person, your doubt should provoke you to investigate the topic of doubt further, at least to prove that you are right in your suspicions. I am saying, very strongly, that you should only doubt any claim if you have constructive arguments to refute the claim.

I firmly believe that a truly educated person is one who has an open mind to the things he or she does not understand and cannot explain. As part of an on-going epistemological enquiry, any speckle or atom of suspicion, doubt or scepticism on a subject of enquiry should give us the green light or the impetus for further investigation in the search for knowledge and certainty in the particular subject of enquiry. This is positive scepticism which leads to further investigation, knowledge and certainty as opposed to plain, naive, doubt which perpetuates ignorance.

You must always remember that until your own investigations, things do not become rubbish, silly or stupid just because you lack the experience or the intellectual ability to understand them! Always remember that what you know is not all there is to know in heaven and earth as William Shakespeare cautions here.

"There are more things in heaven and earth, Horatio,
than are dreamt in your philosophy."
(William Shakespeare, *Hamlet* Act 1, Scene 5)

1.5 Key Points to Remember
There are four levels of mental action.

- ❖ The Conscious level is the level of everyday waking life, the level at which you are reading this book now.
- ❖ The Preconscious level is the level of latent memories which can be recalled at any moment without difficulty.

❖ The Unconscious level is the level of memories which have been repressed and have become inaccessible to the individual.

❖ The Supraconscious level is the level of great natural creativity, inspirational work and the power of the mind for extrasensory perception.

1.6 Belief as an essential ingredient to Stop Smoking

Belief, like action, is an essential ingredient in a recipe for success in anything you do. It is an attitude of mind which encompasses everything you do in relation to the objectives you which to accomplish.

There is an enormous power in believing. A man or woman can achieve a seemingly impossible goal, perform the greatest feat, and achieve a personal best (PB) performance in competitive sports when he or she believes in the possibility of accomplishing the goal. A person's belief or conviction impacts on the way he or she lives his or her life because it can make the difference between success and failure.

You can give up smoking now, easily, and effortlessly if you have a strong belief that you can. Remember the positive possibilities in your journey to the new world in the preparatory exercise at the beginning of this chapter and have the idea of the possibility of success in your mind always.

Belief can be positive or negative. Each form of belief affects the individual differently. A positive belief is a detergent to doubt. A positive belief that you will give up smoking now stirs your mind to positive action and enables you to give up smoking easily, effectively, and effortlessly.

A belief that you would not be able to give up smoking, that it is all a waste of time, is a negative belief. This form of belief blunts the edge of positive action and leaves you incapable of accomplishing your objectives. A negative belief in relation to your goal leads disastrously to failure.

A negative belief fans the flames of doubts and panders to idleness. Both positive and negative beliefs are ways of channelling your energy to your objectives or goals. The positive energies bring success to you while the negative energies bring failure and disappointment to you. To understand this properly, you must refer to the principles of universal energy which I discussed above under the fundamental principles of the power of the mind.

1.7 You Must Have Total Belief and Faith in Yourself

In another sense belief is an attitude of mind which encompasses everything you do in relation to what you wish to achieve. The power of belief is in its usage; it is not something which you possess and leave at home in your briefcase or something which you leave in a box, cupboard, or in your pocket. Belief is something about you which lies in the power within you in expressing your attitudes in everything you do to achieve your objectives. Belief, like confidence, is the way you carry yourself strongly, forcefully, in your actions, attitudes and behaviours from day to day.

There is a strong sense in what I have said above, in which belief refers to absolute trust or confidence. This is the sense in which we use the word **belief** in this book. It is the sense in which someone might say, 'I believe in God' or the sense in which someone might say to another that, 'You must have total belief in yourself'.

This sense of belief is like **faith**, an absolute, confident trust in the truth, value, efficacy, or worthiness of the ideas or plans which you hold on a given project. Belief is, in this sense, very essential for success because it enhances your powers of persistence. You must understand in this sense that no one is ready for success in anything until he or she believes that he or she can acquire it.

You must have absolute faith and trust in yourself and in what you are doing to succeed in your venture. Belief is the opposite of doubt. When you have belief, you pursue your goals without doubting your ability to succeed in them. To understand this much better you must refer to my discussions above on the principles of the power of the mind.

What is pertinent for our present purpose of giving up smoking is that those beliefs which a person, mistakenly, takes as knowledge are recorded permanently in the unconscious mind. These affect the person's attitude in relation to the things that matter in his or her life.

A false and negative belief in relation to giving up smoking and the achievement of success will cause a person to have twisted ideas about giving up smoking. These twisted ideas must be eradicated and replaced with positive ideas backed up with belief for the individual to achieve success with the goal of giving up smoking or with any other goal in a chosen field of endeavour.

Belief is the essential ingredient in a recipe for success in whatever you do. You must have total belief in yourself and in whatever venture you wish to embark on in order to succeed in it. You must have an unwavering, rock solid, absolute belief in yourself and in your ability to give up smoking easily and effortlessly.

Some people start by doubting themselves. They ask, "What if it fails?" They convince themselves that this is an appropriate question. Remember, if you have failure in your mind, that is what you will get. If you are thinking of failure, that will be your reality. Endeavour to think about success in whatever you do, in your goals and aspirations, so that success will be your reality. Refer to the fundamental principles which I discussed above.

1.8 Key Points to Remember

- ❖ Belief is the essential ingredient in a recipe for success in any venture.
- ❖ You must have total belief, a rock solid, absolute faith in yourself to be successful in whatever you do.
- ❖ Belief is the opposite of doubt. When you have belief, you pursue your goals without doubts about your chances of success.
- ❖ Remember that no one is ready for success in anything until he or she believes that he or she can achieve success.

1.9 How to Eliminate the Negative Power of Self Doubt

Remember that belief is the opposite of doubt. Do not defeat yourself by doubting yourself before you start. Do not place unwanted barriers on your path to success through relentless but unnecessary doubts. Self doubt shows insecurity, lack of self esteem and lack of faith in your ability to achieve success with your goal. If you lack faith in yourself, how would you expect others to have faith in you?

The way to get out of the negative, defeatist, thinking trap is to break down the negative thought patterns that restrict you from making essential progress in your chosen field. Whenever negative thoughts flow to your mind in relation to your ability to give up smoking, you must start to cancel them out by thinking positive thoughts about the possibility of attaining your desire of being a non-smoker easily and effectively. Remember your journey to the world of positive possibilities. When you visualize your success, you will be able to realize it, that is, make it real.

You will find that each time you introspect about the good things that have happened to you in your life, all the goals you have achieved in the past till now, or think positive thoughts about your life in general, think about the positive effects of giving up smoking easily, effectively and being a non-smoker right now! If you are unable to visualize, then endeavour to think strong, powerful thoughts about your success in anything you do so that success will be your reality.

You will find that as you concentrate your thoughts in this way, positive feelings will flow, automatically, to you. *Think positive thoughts and positive feelings will flow to you, automatically.* It works every time. Try it **NOW** and see what happens. Go on try it now even as you read this book. You will feel positive instantly. Remember, if you think you can, you will succeed. Think about the positive possibilities of giving up smoking easily, effectively, and effortlessly and you will give up smoking.

If you are disagreeing with me at this moment and saying to yourself that you have not achieved anything in your life, you would be very wrong! Do not be too quick to undermine your achievements or to argue and disagree with me here because this is a sign of your insecurity. Think about it seriously. You may have been quick to disagree with what I have said here because there is anxiety in your life now or, because you have been using the word 'achieve' in a negative sense.

You have achieved some successes in your life. Take a deep breath, through your diaphragm, relax and look back with confidence and you will find plenty of successes in your life. Most important of all, remember that you have conquered some obstacles in life and got over certain difficulties in life to be where you are now.

In addition, you are now making plans for your success with the goal of giving up smoking easily and effectively. You have started on this plan by reading this book and you will finish what you start. Remember the five fundamental principles of the power of the mind which I discussed above. When you believe in yourself and think positive thoughts in the way that I am teaching you here, things will happen for you as you wish them to happen. They happen because you are making them happen by the effective use of the power within you.

Begin **today** to develop a different sense of value about yourself, self-worth, time, energy, work, and your desire to give up smoking. Begin from now onwards to evaluate yourself positively, to project a positive self image. Begin now to believe in yourself for this will help you to give up smoking easily and effectively.

If you hold negative beliefs about yourself, about the idea of success in giving up smoking, then the thing to do now is to change your pattern of beliefs and begin today to see that success is within your grasp because the magic power of success is within you. Start from now to believe in yourself and you will easily see a way out of any difficult situation.

Start from now to believe that there is **always** a way out of any problem. Begin now to do things differently from the way you have done in the past. This is what making a change is about, doing something new or at least different from before. Start from today to believe that life is full of doors of opportunities which are coming to you. Believe it for it is true. You will find them when you seek for them.

Use your mind positively to find a way out of any current problem which you may have. If you want to make progress in the face of mounting problems, remember to *always look on the bright side of life* and then do something new or, at least, different from what you have done in the past. This book offers you something different, new methods of dealing with problems through mental action. Your mind is the very fertile womb through which all the thoughts for positive mental constructions are incubated and hatched.

1.10 Key Points to Remember

* ❖ Remember that whenever you think positive thoughts about yourself, your goals and aspirations, you will find that positive feelings flow to you automatically.
* ❖ Always look on the bright side of life because irrational negativism dampens the spirits of positive action.
* ❖ Remember that belief is a detergent to doubt.

1.11 Positive Strategies to Enhance Your Success in Giving up Smoking

How to Guard Against Negatives in General

For an individual to achieve success in whatever venture he or she embarks on, he or she must endeavour to guard himself or herself against negative influences. Some negative influences may be of the individual's own making. Where this is the case, it is often difficult for the individual to recognise the negative influences upon him or her because people, in general, do not perceive themselves as impediments to their own progress.

Other negative influences may be the result of the activities of the negative people with whom the individual associates, that is, the company he or she keeps or the negative environment in which he or she works in or lives in. If you live or work with people who influence you to smoke against your wishes you must begin from now to tell them that you are now a non-smoker. To gather the confidence to take control and dispel the negative influence of other people, you must make the journey to the world of positive possibilities now. Refer to the beginning of this chapter.

Whatever the nature of the negative influences in an individual's life, and whatever form they have been derived, the individual must be able to recognise these negative influences and eliminate them. The elimination of the negative influences will enhance the individual's ability to feel mentally free to entertain positive thoughts about success. This is particularly relevant in giving up smoking because friends and associates may attempt to deter one from a chosen purpose by their negative vibrations. Concentrate on your plans and you will be successful with your goal to stop smoking easily and effectively.

An individual must become aware of his or her own will power and remember, always, that the magic of success is truly within him or her. The recognition of this will alert the person to the power of the unconscious mind and thus help him or her to eliminate negatives from his or her thoughts in relation to the goal to stop smoking. An individual must become aware that negative thoughts will affect him or her if such thoughts take hold in his or her unconscious mind.

In this respect, it is most appropriate for an individual to avoid the association of people whose company drain the individual's energy psychically and makes the individual feel low, depressed, or unhappy in some ways. If you wish to stop smoking now, easily, and effortlessly you must avoid the association of negative people who constantly make you feel bad by making you to smoke against your will.

To eliminate such negatives influences a person must master the five fundamental principles of the power of the mind which I discussed above because a sound knowledge of the five fundamental principles is a detergent to negative influences. An individual must also seek the company of people in whose association he or she gets an uplift, people who inspire him or her with confidence and make him or her feel good about himself or herself, or people whose achievements he or she admires and seeks to emulate.

1.12 Confront Your Fear to Conquer It

Do not be afraid of success. Some individuals are afraid of success but they convince themselves that they are afraid of failure so they fail to act on opportunities that come their way and, thus, fail to accomplish their objective just as they fail to recognize their own negative thinking. When you say that you are afraid of 'failure', you concentrate on 'failure' and, so 'failure' becomes your reality.

If you are seeking to achieve success then, you should never think of 'failure' because it is a negation of what you are seeking. Do not be afraid of success. Do not think that you will fail because if you think of failure, failure will become your reality. Remember the five fundamental principles discussed in this chapter. If you are thinking of failure, this will become your reality. You must confront your fear in order to conquer it.

Fear is a negative emotion which is an impediment to your goal to stop smoking and it can be manifested by your vacillation, procrastination and doubting your own ability to succeed with your goal to stop smoking. Sometimes people vacillate and procrastinate because they are uncertain of what to do and this uncertainty may be the result of insecurity which, also, leads to fear. Thus, here, there is a circle which can be a vicious circle in certain individual circumstances.

Fear is a hindrance to success in general and must be confronted for the individual to succeed in a chosen goal. Many sporting personalities and teams have lost competitions because they were afraid of the opponents. Think about success in giving up smoking so that success will become your reality.

Fear is ordinarily an emotional or physiological response to a consciously recognized source of danger. The normal response takes the form of voluntary avoidance of the feared object. However, fear can occur unconsciously and may be employed by a person in a defence mechanism as a pretext to exculpate the failure to act in a certain way. Instances of such defences may occur if the person concerned has convinced himself or herself that he or she is afraid of attempting to stop smoking.

In such circumstances, such a person, then, automatically avoids anything that will lead him or her to attempt to stop smoking. Thus, he or she never takes part in any ventures to do with stop smoking because of his or her fear. The effect of such fear is that it destroys positive thoughts about the goal to stop smoking, weakens the power of reflection on the advantages of the goal to stop smoking and discourages positive effort in relation to stop smoking in general and leads, inexorably, to failure.

Remember my discussions above about the powers of the unconscious mind. You will understand from this that fear will have a very dangerous effect on a person's attempt to stop smoking. As I have described above, if a person is afraid of doing something, the natural response is to avoid the object or topic of fear.

In doing so, the fear and the act of avoidance are retained in the unconscious. This results in negative thinking. The individual becomes afraid and believes that to stop smoking will be a difficult task to accomplish. He or she becomes afraid to attempt the task because of the negative belief.

Thus, when a person gives expression to fear in the form of negative and destructive thoughts about stop smoking, he or she is very likely to experience the result of the fear in the form of destructive repercussions. The negative thoughts are retained in the unconscious and this becomes part of his or her general attitude, response, reaction, and behavioural traits in relation to stop smoking. Such a person becomes a very negative, fearful, cowardly person lacking courage and moral fibre to make a definite decision to stop smoking and stick with the decision or to embark on anything worthwhile because of fear.

If a person wishes to stop smoking and, at the same time, has a fear of the goal to stop smoking, fears that he or she might fail to stop smoking, then it is clear from my discussion of fear here, that such a person has a psychological conflict. Such conflict is necessary in the development of neurotic anxiety and all those seemingly simple problems that blight an individual's enjoyment of everyday life. For a fuller discussion of **conflicts** in the development of psychoneurotic problems, refer to my book, (Maurice-Nneke, 2003).

There are two general fears that people have which, depending on the affect on the person, might deter efforts to make progress with the goal to stop smoking. These fears are, generally, anxiety that something will go wrong in whatever the individual wishes to do. Thus, to prevent it from going wrong, the individual does not carry out the intended action or venture. It becomes a great anxiety problem when the individual begins to expect things to go wrong and feels disappointed, angry, and frustrated when things do not wrong when he or she attempts to carry out the action.

Anticipated traumatic stress disorder (**ATSD**) is one of such fears where the individual has the expectation that something will go wrong at anytime on any venture. This is the result of insecurity, self-doubt, and an inability to feel adequate in any role or in any activity that one engages in, including the appoint to meet a stranger at any environment.

Some smokers also appeal to **Murphy's Law** and assure themselves that it is a natural law to the effect that anything that can go wrong will go wrong. As the anxiety of ATSD, Murphy's Law concentrates on the negation of what the individual wishes to achieve. It is boosted by self-doubt and negative thoughts.

Think positive thoughts about your goal to stop smoking and everything will go right for you. Try to remember your journey to the world of positive possibility and enact the journey until you feel confident enough to carry on with your goal to stop smoking.

1.13 How to Deal with the Effects of Stress, Anxiety and Depression (SAD)

The effects of stress, anxiety, and psychological depression can be very damaging to a person's personality. They can lead to apathy, lack of confidence and very low self-esteem. Thus, stress, anxiety and psychological depression bring about destructive negative attitudes which are barriers to progress in a chosen goal such as stop smoking. Indeed, for some individuals, stress, anxiety, and psychological depression may be the cause of their smoking problem.

The people who suffer from anxiety problems, those who live or work in stressful environment or those who suffer from psychological depression, find it difficult to live in a healthy way. They may smoke constantly for comfort and thus may convince themselves that smoking helps them to feel relaxed.

The reality is that excessive smoking for comfort makes the individual tense, nervous and irritable. This is the effect of the mass of tar and nicotine in the individual's metabolic system. I use the term, *psychological depression,* to refer to an emotional problem of interpersonal relations which leads to a deep feeling of unhappiness and total inadequacy. This is distinguished from *organic depression* which is the result of some injury to the brain.

The unhappiness involved in psychological depression is often manifested in the individual's need to resort to food, alcohol, or cigarette as a means of comfort but the reality of the situation is that it is a means of escape for the individual. That is, to say, the individual is running away from the need to confront the problem.

For some other people suffering from stress, anxiety and psychological depression, food, alcohol and cigarettes offer a means of denial of their problem. They act as a defence mechanism since for such people, the enjoyment of food, alcohol and cigarettes give the illusory feeling that everything is fine with them, that they are relaxed as I have mentioned above.

A person who suffers from psychological depression has certain underlying psychological problems which make him or her feel very low and unhappy. As I have mentioned above, where certain underlying feeling of unhappiness exists in an individual's life, it is often difficult for the individual to attend positively to a goal such as giving up smoking.

Such a person, usually, resorts to negative attitudes such as self-pity, excuses, etc. Stress, anxiety and psychological depression are barriers to giving of smoking because they prevent an individual from concentrating fully on the tasks and exercises that are conducive to the goal to stop smoking easily, effectively and effortlessly.

To find out whether you are properly attuned in your mind to the goal to stop smoking easily and effectively, you must examine your private life thoroughly and answer the following questions truthfully and honestly to yourself.

- ❖ Do you have stress and anxiety in your life?
- ❖ Do you suffer from episodes of depression in your life?
- ❖ Are you depressed now?
- ❖ Are you prone to destructive negative thoughts most of the time?
- ❖ Do you live with people or a person who abuse you, bully or beat you?

Do not be troubled because it is not an intelligent test or an aptitude test. However, if you are frank and sincere in your answers you will find out more about your own personal issues and then be able to make improvements as necessary. If you admit to anxiety and depression, it is best that you deal with these problems first by consulting your own physician who may be able to recommend a psychotherapist.

You will find that the solution of the problems will enable you to concentrate more on your chosen venture of giving up smoking, easily and effectively. Here are the rest of the exercises which you must now administer to yourself before I take you through some essential exercises which will help you to stop smoking.

1.14 Examining Your Level of Stress, Anxiety, and Depression
Recognising the SAD Effect
A person who is afflicted with stress, anxiety, and depression is very usually a sad person. The sadness is often noticed in his or her behaviour and attitudes by other people with whom he or she comes into contact such as family, friends or working colleagues. By coincidence, the first letters of the words *stress, anxiety, depression,* spell out **SAD** just as in the case of the condition known as *seasonal affective disorder.*

Stress gives rise to tension which creates conflict to the existing situation. This makes the individual to be unease, that is, dis-eased. Thus, the individual has an illness. This is shown by the anxiety and depression which are treatable illnesses. Now, you can see the connections, if you do not know them before.

Find out whether this **SAD** effect is part of your personal issue or whether it is implicated in your behaviour or in your everyday attitudes towards people or things and events around you.

Answer the following questions in your own way but truthfully to yourself. If you choose to answer just 'YES' or 'NO' to any of the questions, let your 'YES' or 'NO' be represented by what happens to you most of the time with the situation described in the questions. Do not say 'It depends on...' as an answer to any of the question because the questions concern general situations, not contextual or private circumstances or situations in your life.

However, if you choose to answer 'YES' or 'NO' to any questions, be particularly careful that you do not answer 'YES' and 'NO' to the same question. For example, in the third question below, if your general attitude is to interrupt when people talk with you, then your answer to the question would be 'YES'. If you are unable to decide what your answer to a question should be and if you think that the questions are designed to annoy you or make you reveal your deep secrets, this is indicative that there are, indeed, certain underlying problems in your life.

If any of the questions make you say to yourself, "Everyone does that", you will be wrong because you do not **know** *everyone* however much you may wish to think that you do! At the best, all the people you know may be doing that, but all the people that you know are not, strictly speaking, *everyone*. They are just *some* people that do whatever is implied in the question. In matters such as those in the questions, it is best to speak for yourself always but not for everyone. The questions require you to speak for yourself.

By saying to yourself or to others that "Everyone does that" you are, unconsciously, employing the psychological defence mechanism of *rationalisation*. You are trying to make your unwanted behaviour or habit 'fit' with what you think everyone does, that is, you imply that you are the same as everyone. This is to show that all is well with you since your habit, action or behaviour is in accord with public habit, action, or behaviour. By doing this, you are defending yourself already before anyone has accused you of anything!

Just relax and remember that your name does not appear anywhere on the questions. They are general, questions and you are reading them alone in your own privacy and giving the answers to yourself. There is, therefore, nothing to be alarmed about. Now, read carefully and answer all the questions sincerely and honestly to yourself in your own way.

1. In general, are you a negative or a positive person?
2. Would you describe yourself as an optimist or a pessimist?
3. Do you often interrupt when someone is talking to you?
4. Are you always in a rush but, really, not accomplishing anything?
5. Can you wait your turn patiently?
6. Do you usually hide your feelings?
7. Do you do lots of things at once?
8. Would you describe yourself as a difficult person?
9. Do you often feel you want to burst into tears?
10. Do you bite your nails?
11. Do you have any nervous twitches?
12. Do you find it hard to concentrate or make decisions?
13. Do you often feel irritable, snappy, or unfriendly?
14. Do you often find yourself eating when you are not hungry?
15. Do you regularly drink or smoke to calm your nerves?
16. Do you sleep badly?
17. Have you lost interest in sex?
18. Do you feel increasingly gloomy and suspicious of other people?
19. Do you blush when people look straight at you?
20. Are you a calm person who is not easily upset?
21. Can you sit still without fidgeting?
22. Can you keep your cool when your plans fail to work?
23. Are you afraid of the dark?
24. Are you afraid of death?
25. Are you afraid of cancer?
26. Are you afraid of blood?
27. Are you afraid of heights?
28. Have you ever used tranquillisers to calm your nerves?
29. Are you on tranquillisers now?
30. Do you care about making an impression by what you do?
31. Do you often stop to examine your motives?

32. *Do you care much about what other people think of you?*
33. *Do you seem to have more than your share of bad luck?*
34. *Do you feel usually depressed when you wake up in the morning?*
35. *In general are you satisfied with your life so far?*
36. *Do you often suffer from loneliness?*
37. *Do you consider your future as quite bright?*

1.15 Examining Whether You Are in Control

1. *Are there some habits of yours that you would like to break but cannot?*
2. *Do you make your decisions despite what other people concerned have to say?*
3. *If something you have planned goes wrong, do you usually admit it is your own fault rather than blame it on bad luck?*
4. *Do you often feel that you are the victim of other peoples plots or outside forces which you cannot control?*
5. *Are you always persuaded into action by what other people say?*
6. *Do you believe that it is possible for a person to change his/her personality?*
7. *Do you reckon that you can do things as well as other people?*
8. *Do you spend more of your time thinking about success or failure?*
9. *Do you sometimes think about yourself as a failure?*
10. *Are there many things about yourself that you would like to change if you could?*
11. *Are you bothered by other people's criticisms of your personality or your actions?*
12. *Do you often think that other people are better liked than yourself?*
13. *Can you honestly say that you rarely feel ashamed of anything you have done?*
14. *Do you often set your aspirations low in order to avoid disappointments?*
15. *Do you try to do things immediately rather than put them off until later?*
16. *Do you always try to finish the things you start?*
17. *Do you always tend to be jealous or envious of the success of other people?*

18. Have you ever felt that you would really like to kill someone?

19. If someone does you a bad turn do you usually ignore it?

20. Do you sometimes get so annoyed that you break crockery or throw things around the house?

21. Do you usually resort to tantrums as your only way of attracting attention to ourselves?

1.16 Examining Your Power to Project Yourself Positively

1. Do you usually seek revenge when someone hurts you in any way?

2. Would you rather agree with what someone had said to avoid an argument?

3. Do you feel that if someone is rude to you it is best to ignore them and let the occasion pass?

4. Do you often make sarcastic remarks about other people in their presence or behind their back?

5. Do you tolerate negative or discouraging influences which you can easily avoid?

6. If you have been waiting on a queue for a long time and someone came in and went straight to the front of the queue would you do something about it?

7. Do you usually put yourself second in matters relating to your family?

8. Do you believe that it is necessary to fight for your rights or else you lose them?

9. Do you complain if something you purchased in good faith turns out to be a fake?

10. You were ignored in a store. Do you act to attract attention or just leave quietly?

1.17 Key Points to Remember

- ❖ Always guard against negative thoughts and endeavour to be positive at least, most of the time.
- ❖ Endeavour to eliminate the SAD effect, if any, from your life.
- ❖ Take control of your life and project yourself positively.

CHAPTER TWO: THE GOAL AND A PLAN OF ACTION TO STOP SMOKING

You will get what you want for what you want is what you get

2.1 Introduction

A prime requisite for success is to determine accurate goals or objectives. This is accomplished by establishing what you regard as your major and minor goals. A major goal may be something which would bring a major change in an individual's life or it may be those objectives which the individual hopes to achieve within a long period of time, for example, say within three years, five years, ten years, etc. as in the expressed desire, *'By this time in five years I will be a billionaire!'*

A minor goal should be a range of objectives which a person seeks to achieve this month, within the next three months or within the next six months. In certain cases, there may be a series of minor goals leading to the fulfilment of a major goal.

In this case, the goal to stop smoking now is a shot term goal because it needs to be fulfilled now. However, it can be a major goal for an individual if attaining the desired smoke free life style involves a major goal of the individual or if the attainment of the desired non-smoker status would bring a major change in the individual's life. Nevertheless, the time element *'Now'* in the goal and in the title of this book is indicative of the urgency of the wish and the necessity to accomplish it immediately or within a short time.

2.2 How to Formulate the Goal to Stop Smoking Now!

For the specific purpose here, to stop smoking now, a well formulated goal must have the following characteristics.

1. The Goal must be specific and Clearly Defined.
Every individual has a series of ambitions, desires, hopes, needs, wants, wishes. These, initially, are not goals but each one of your ambitions,

desires, hopes, needs, wants, or wishes can become your major goal or minor goal from the moment the ambition, desire, hope, need, want, or wish is isolated from the rest and made the central focus of your mental and physical energy, that is the energy required for your mental and physical efforts to achieve the objective. Refer to the third principle discussed above in the first chapter of this book.

To isolate any objective and make it into a goal you must put your series of ambitions, desires, hopes, needs, wants, and wishes into a scale of relative preference and deal with the one that is most pressing, most urgent, or most easily attainable. You must deal with the economic consideration involved. For example, the most pressing and most urgent objective may not be the most easily achievable.

Something becomes a goal for an individual when, after all the work of consideration and deliberations in evaluating its merits and disadvantages, the individual isolates it from the series of other ambitions, desires, needs, wants, or wishes, etc, which are open to him or her, and then focus all mental and physical energies towards achieving that objective.

For example, to achieve the goal to stop smoking easily and effortlessly, the individual can focus his or her attention on the health and integrity of his or her body, the need to get back the strength and stamina which was lost through smoking, the need for positive thoughts about himself or herself and his or her ability to succeed in the goal. He or she must have self belief. Remember that no one is ready for success in any goal unless he or she believes that he or she can achieve success in the goal.

Defining your goal clearly means that it should be properly distinguished from your range of other interests, ambitions, desires, need, wants, and wishes. It also means that the road to the fulfilment of your goal must be clearly mapped out showing what you ought to do, the length of time you have set aside to do it, and how you are to do what you ought to do to achieve the goal. In other words, defining the goal entails part of the action plan to accomplish the goal

2. The Goal must involve new Behaviour or new Activity and a Plan of Action

When a goal is clearly formulated the formulation will include the definition of what the goal entails, and the plan of action that would bring the goal about. The execution of this plan must involve the individual in new behaviours, doing things which he or she has not done before or things which he or she is not doing now.

Thus, to achieve the goal the individual must be actively involved in a new form of activity or behaviour. To stop smoking easily and effortlessly the individual must start with a new course of action such as the regime of mental action which this book brings to you.

3. The Goal must be Positive and Realistic

If your goals are positive, they become easy for you to fulfil and you will fulfil them much quicker if they are realistic. The goal to stop smoking is a positive goal for an individual in respect of the improvement to the person's health. The person gains also in strength, energy, stamina and vitality which an individual derives from the cessation of the debilitation effect of smoking.

4. The Goal must be Available

If you have taken great care and thought to formulate and define your goal you will see, easily, that if the goal is within your reaches, it will be attainable effortlessly. At one of my *Self Help Workshops* a gentleman participant stated that his goal was to own a Rolls Royce car. As he had no savings and investments and was earning only £100 per week from his employment at the time you can see, quite clearly, that the stated goal was not available to him at the time.

There is every reason to say that, although the goal was a positive one in so far as it was forward looking, it was indeed an unrealistic goal in respect of his financial position at the time. It is obvious that in view of his financial position the desire (for it was only a desire for him at the time not a goal yet!) for a Rolls Royce car will take an awfully long time to be accomplished. Thus, his immediate goal would, more appropriately, be a change of employment to a higher wage structure.

The goal to stop smoking can be an available goal to any individual in respect of the details of his or her health if he or she is in a fit and proper condition to participate fully in all the practical exercises in this book.

5. The Goal must be Located in the Individual's Environment
The goal must be within your own environment or situation. For example, if a person's goal is to be Prime Minister it follows that to achieve the goal, he or she must be a politician or else he or she never gets to achieve such a goal in a democratic country. The method of achieving a political goal by buying one's way into high office or just seize power by armed means is, generally, not the normal way to accomplish or fulfil a political goal.

As in my illustration above, to be Prime Minister of a democratic nation like the United Kingdom, for instance, a person must be in politics and win his or her seat in a general election. He or she must also be the leader of the party that won the general election or be the winner of a party leadership contest by challenging the incumbent Prime Minister directly, or the winner of a leadership election in the event of a resignation or death of a Prime Minister.

What is relevant from these illustrations is that being a politician in a democratic country places the individual in a situation from which he or she can fulfil a goal of being Prime Minister. However, a British politician whose goal is to be the President of the USA would be setting his or her goal far beyond his or her environment. Thus, he or she will be making it too difficult or relatively impossible to fulfil for him or her to fulfil the goal.

However, I must acknowledge the fact that there have been some Presidents of the USA who won the presidency without having held political office previously. These include Donald Trump (2017-2021), Dwight D. Eisenhower (1953-1961), Herbert Hoover (1929-1933), Ulysses S. Grant (1869-1877), and Zachary Taylor (1849-1850). The most recent president without a political background was Donald Trump who was a businessman and television personality.

We would say from the above illustrations that the goal to stop smoking is ordinarily within the environment of any individual since to stop smoking entails what one does to oneself. However, the method by which an individual chooses to do this might be stringent and thus, remote to the individual's metabolism.

The method that I advocate in this book is positive thoughts about one's goals and aspirations. It is mental and so it is within the environment of any individual who can use his or her mind profitably in positive thoughts.

6. The Goal must be kept constantly in Mind
Remember from what I said above about the unconscious mind that your ideas must be clearly imprinted and fully developed in your mind for them to work for you. When you have taken the time and mental energy to formulate your goal, define it clearly and plan the action for its fulfilment, it becomes necessary that you must keep the goal constantly in your mind to fulfil it.

It can be seen from this, that the failure of an individual to keep the goal constantly in the mind may result in the individual forgetting the goal completely or replacing it with other desires on his or her scale of preference. In the methods which I advocate in this book, the goal to stop smoking is a goal of mental action so it is much more amenable to be kept in the mind.

2.3 How to Define Your Goal
Your goal must be stated clearly and precisely. One needs to be very specific in defining a goal. This is very important so that the action plans for achieving the goal are specifically directed and the mind is clearly focused on the goal. Your knowledge of the functions of the unconscious mind which I discussed above will help you to understand the need to be clear and specific in your definition of the goal.

The aim here is to fulfil your desire to stop smoking now and to do so easily, completely, and effectively. Notice that the element of time is already entailed by our title, *'Stop Smoking Now!'* Thus, you can define the goal in the following terms and this will also form part of your relaxation exercise. In this way, the goal will be firmly established in your mind.

Your goal is to stop smoking now and to do so completely, easily, effectively and to remain a non-smoker from this moment onwards. The goal to stop smoking, completely, easily, and effectively will fill you with pleasure and happiness. You will feel the sensation of pleasure as you begin to breathe clearly and have more strength, energy, and stamina day by day in every way.

You will regard each clear breath that you take as a sign of the success of your action plan and you will be very happy knowing that with each passing day from this moment onwards you are concerned more and more for the general improvement of the health and integrity of your body.

You will be totally relaxed and completely in control from this moment onwards because you know that you will achieve success with your goal to stop smoking now! When you stop smoking completely, easily, and effectively and continue to be relaxed everyday you will find that the feeling of total relaxation, the feeling of being in control, the feeling of peace of mind and general well-being will stay with you and become part of your everyday feelings from this moment onwards.

You will be confident, positive, and optimistic in your outlook and you will love yourself because of the success you are achieving with your goal. From this moment, onwards as you continue to feel positive and happy, you will be able to show a positive attitude of love towards the people that matter in your life and you do this by your faithful adherence to your goal to stop smoking now and stop forcing them to become passive smokers by smoking around them.

The above is the goal clearly defined. This must be stated clearly and distinctly so that the unconscious mind understands your intention in relation to your goal to stop smoking (or whatever goal you might have). If the above definition of your goal is chosen it indicates to the unconscious mind that you want to stop smoking completely, easily, and effectively as I stated above. In this way, the unconscious mind will help you to accomplish your goal easily and effortlessly.

Gaining Access to the Unconscious mind through Deep Relaxation
Now that your goal is clearly defined, you must induce yourself into a state of deep relaxation to gain access to the unconscious mind. You must begin with the following procedure.

How to induce yourself into a state of Deep Relaxation
Settle down and make yourself comfortable on a chair, couch or on the floor. Now, take a deep breath, long and slow, through your diaphragm. Hold your breath for a mental count of 5, or 10 (or whatever number that is suitable for you), exhale gently and allow the air to spread through your body as you R E L A X. Repeat this three, or four times (or as many times as it is possible to loosen yourself up).

Now imagine yourself out in the open air. Make it a beautiful place and a beautiful day just as you would like it to be. You may choose to be on a sandy beach, in a park or even in your back garden. Wherever it is that you've chosen to be at this moment in your mind, make it a place which represents for you the very ultimate in peace, joy and total relaxation.

As you continue to relax this way from day to day you will find that you will feel very peaceful with each passing day. This feeling of peace and total relaxation will become a part of the way you feel from day to day. This feeling will become an attitude of mind and body for you. You will be very profoundly relaxed in mind and body wherever you happen to be and whatever the situation or the circumstances in which you find yourself. You will be absolutely relaxed and in control come what may.

Relaxation will give you the peace of mind and the inner tranquillity which enables you to deal with any situation that you come across and helps you to take complete control of your life.

Now allow the feeling of relaxation to surge through every part of your body more and more. Begin from the top of your head and feel your scalp and your forehead relaxing, feel the muscles around your eyes relax, feel your cheeks and the muscles around your mouth relax, feel the whole of your face relax.

This feeling of relaxation begins now to spread down from your face to your neck and throat and from there it spreads across your shoulders and from your shoulders through your arms to the tips of your fingers with your wrists and your elbows very deeply relaxed. Concentrate now on your chest and your upper back and feel relaxation spreading from your chest to your abdomen and from your upper back to your lower back so the trunk of your body is very deeply relaxed.

Now feel your waist and your bottom relax. This feeling of relaxation spreads to your pelvis, then your thighs, and from your thighs all the way through your knees and your lower legs to the tips of your toes. Your entire body relaxes. Now feel relaxation surging through your body from the top of your head to the tips of your toes and from the tips of your toes to the top of your head.

As you continue to relax this way, you will find that the stress and the strain of the day will go out of your mind and out of your body. With increased relaxation, you can let go your worries and your anxieties and allow the feeling of peace and inner calmness into your body and into your life.

You are now feeling a deep, profound relaxation in every part of your body, every fibre, every atom, and every particle of your body. Your entire body is now deeply relaxed and serene. With this relaxation, you should feel peaceful and comfortable and as you become totally relaxed and completely in control, you may experience either a tingling sensation spreading through your body, or a feeling of lightness, or weightlessness as if you are about to fly away on your own, or a combination of those feelings.

As you are now deeply relaxed your unconscious mind is ready to receive positive instructions for your present and future well-being, for your happiness and to enable you to stop smoking now, easily, and effectively.

Note: As you are now deeply relaxed, your unconscious mind is now ready to receive positive instructions or mental prompts for your present and future well-being, for your happiness and to enable you to stop smoking now, steadily, easily, and effectively. This note can also be incorporated in your relaxation technique as I have done it above thus allowing your goal to stop smoking now, easily, and effectively to be imprinted on your unconscious mind and become easily achievable by you.

The effect of this will be lasting for you because as your goal is imprinted in your unconscious mind your motor activities will reflect it. In this way, the actions which will lead to the fulfilment of your goal will become part of your everyday motor activities. Refer to the fundamental principles of the mind technique in chapter one.

Positive Instructions or Mental Prompts
When you have attained a deep level of relaxation you can then give yourself positive instructions in relation to your desired goal which you have previously defined. These instructions will, indeed, be a repetition of the essential details of your goal as I have defined it, above. I have defined a goal for stop smoking now, above.

Now for further illustration, let us suppose that you have another goal which is to eliminate pain from your body. Let us make it more interesting and suppose, further, that it is the elimination of period pains, pain of arthritis or pain during childbirth. Let us settle for pain during childbirth. Male readers may concentrate on the pain of arthritis or any other pain they may have. We may begin as follows.

From this moment, onwards when you use the word R E L A X, you will immediately feel as relaxed, comfortable, and serene as you are now. The word R E L A X will mean complete calm, peace, confidence, and total tranquillity in your entire being. When the contractions begin during the birth of your baby the word R E L A X will turn the contractions to pleasurable sensations within your body and you will feel calm and confident.

You will be serene and anaesthetised to the contractions while enjoying happy, pleasurable, sensations in your body. These pleasurable sensations are a sign that your baby is about to arrive. The sign of the arrival of your baby fills you with great joy.

*As you are relaxed, you will be in total control throughout the birth because of your confidence and your knowledge that you have the **inner power to switch off** any unwanted sensation in your body. You will be full of joy, full of energy and vitality. The contractions will give you a feeling of joy. You will feel joy in the knowledge that your baby is about to arrive and the contractions are necessary for the arrival of your baby. You will feel pleasure as your baby enters the birth canal and each movement in your body gives you a pleasurable sensation in the knowledge that the waiting is all over and your baby is about to emerge.*

The feeling of calm and confidence, joy and happiness will continue for you well after the birth of your baby and you will be always relaxed and in control, calm, full of confidence and contentment, full of energy and vitality day by day in every way. The birth of your baby will be a satisfying, pleasurable experience. You will feel totally relaxed and confident and you will show great love and affection for your baby and exhibit a positive attitude of love towards all your dear ones.

Note:

Notice that I have used some of the positive expressions that I used at the preparatory exercises in chapter one. This is for familiarity. Your mind is already familiar with these positive words and will react to them positively when you focus your mind clearly on your objective. In this exercise, if you cannot remember the essential details of your goal, use a summary that contains the gist of what you want to achieve. Always use positive expressions and avoid the temptation to use negative terms.

Always affirm the things that you want to achieve not their negation. Here is an example of a positive affirmation.

"During the birth of my baby I will feel a pleasurable sensation in my body and I will feel calm, confident, totally relaxed and absolutely in control".

In contrast to the example above, consider the following statement as an affirmation.

"During the birth of my baby I will not panic, and I will not feel any pain".

The above statement is an emphasis on what the individual will not do. The emphasis must always be on what the individual will do. The above statement is, therefore, a negative and dangerous affirmation in so far as it is focused on panic and pain. These are feelings which the expectant mother does not want during the birth of her baby. You must always be on your guard against the temptation to make such dangerous affirmation.

Note that I have used the pain of childbirth here. This is merely for the illustration. Remember that the gist of the mental prompts in my illustration can be applied to your goal to stop smoking now and to remain as a non-smoker always and be able to feel good, generally.

The above procedure is what you need for your goal to stop smoking now. However, you will learn more techniques in the next chapter so that you have the option to choose the method that suits you best.

2.4 Key Point to Remember
 - ❖ It is necessary to be deeply relaxed in mind and body to bring about the desired changes.

Now, I will show you how everything that I have said here about goals fits in with an individual's actual problems and the goal to stop smoking.

2.5 Problem: The 60 Cigarettes a Day Smoker
A disturbed man gave the following information about himself and his problem.

I am 45 years old and I have been a smoker for 30 years. I smoke cigarettes, not pipe. I smoke first thing in the morning and I smoke in bed too. I smoke after I have had a meal and I smoke cigarettes whenever I have any drinks such as alcohol, coffee, or tea. Whatever drink I have, I smoke with it by force of habit. But I do not really enjoy it because smoking leaves a bad taste in my mouth.

I smoke because I cannot help it, I have got to smoke or I'll have nothing. I am addicted to smoking and I think I am obsessed with the thoughts of smoking.

It is something I must do to keep me going. Sometimes I cough heavily when I smoke and I have recently noticed that I am now coughing constantly as I have bouts of coughing every day, but I notice this in other people too so I do not worry about the cough.

I feel stressed and stretched out from day to day and I have no strength or energy for anything. I am always tired. I have been insulted often by people who tell me that I reek of smoke and that I have bad breath and, although I do not notice these things, they have begun to bother me seriously and I really want to stop smoking now.

2.6 Stop Smoking Now! Goal: To Stop Smoking NOW!

What will it take to have a successful stop smoking programme? It will take seriousness and a defined goal as I have shown you above on 2.3. The formula for this can be stated as follows. CDG + SAP = SSSP, where CDG is *clearly defined goal,* SAP is *serious action plan,* and SSSP is *successful stop smoking programme.*

Remember that we are dealing with **the power of the mind,** how you can use the thinking power of your mind to achieve your goals successfully or how those who are negatively inclined can prevent themselves from achieving a desired success by their negative thoughts.

If you have followed the discussions here attentively you would be able to see quite easily, clearly, the power of the gentleman's negative thoughts. By using your mind solely for negative thoughts, you would be eliminating yourself from the benefits of the opportunities around you and, thus, preventing yourself from achieving the success that you would, otherwise, have enjoyed, yet blaming your failure on other people!

In the case of the *60 Cigarettes a Day Smoker* his addiction to smoking tendencies and negative thinking were preventing him from an attempt to stop smoking and enjoy good health with strength and energy. It is obvious that he wants to stop smoking because the insults of other people have begun to bother him. His problem is introduced here as a *complaint.*

This indicates that the current situation is an unwanted situation, perhaps it is an intolerable situation. However, he postpones the attempt to take positive action to deal with the situation by saying that he cannot help it because smoking is something he must do to keep him going. He also tells us that he must smoke or he will have nothing.

Now in making those statements as his reasons for smoking, he makes out that smoking is necessary for his life and, unconsciously, plays the *self pity* card which, in this instance, is a defence mechanism against taking a positive action to look after his health by taking precautions against the poison of further smoking.

This form of defence is known as *rationalisation.* It sounds good on the surface but deep down it prevents the individual from taking positive action on any uncomfortable or unwanted situation. The *60 Cigarettes a Day Smoker* takes his stated reason for smoking to be an affirmation of truth and so does nothing about it.

This is, indeed, his problem. He is affirming what he does not want, that is, affirming the negation of what he really wants. So, he gets what he affirms because this is what has been imprinted on the unconscious mind. His negative thinking provides him with an excuse for not bothering to take care of his general health and wellbeing.

There is, therefore, a conflict which is what is making it difficult for him to see the actual problem and, then, stop smoking. The conflict is between his unexpressed wish to stop smoking because it is dangerous to his health and his expressed belief that he must continue to smoke because it is what keeps him going. He must resolve this conflict to stop smoking completely, easily, and effortlessly. He must remember that *there is always a way out of any problem* through the positive use of the powers of the mind.

With the idea of positive thoughts in mind, let us now turn the *60 Cigarettes a Day Smoker's* desire to stop smoking now into a goal to stop smoking now with the incentive of regaining his strength, energy, and stamina, become fit and healthy and free from embarrassing cough and see how a positive frame of mind will help him to fulfil his desire.

This positive frame of mind will be implicated in his beliefs, attitudes, the way he channels his energy and it is best described in an *action plan*.

2.7 How to Make an Action Plan for the Goal: To Stop Smoking NOW!
The fulfilment of any goal requires a positive frame of mind which is defined in an action plan. An *Action Plan* is a definite plan of action, activities or tasks which must be performed in order to accomplish the goal. It sets out the course of actions, sets out the various actions which are necessary for the fulfilment of the desired goal. For the stated goal on behalf of the *60 Cigarettes a Day Smoker*, the necessary actions and attitudes must include action to eliminate smoking odour and action to improve strength and energy. The action plan can be stated as follows.

2.8 Action Plan 1: Expressing Self Belief
- ❖ I can stop smoking completely, easily, and effectively because I believe that I have the power to do so.
- ❖ I can stop smoking completely, easily, and effectively because that is my goal.
- ❖ I can stop smoking completely, easily, and effectively because I am concerned for my health.
- ❖ I believe that I am a very determined man who sets goals and fulfils them.
- ❖ I believe that I can be a non-smoker because that is what I want.
- ❖ I am a sociable person and I believe that smoking is now an anti-social behaviour.
- ❖ I firmly believe that the Hollywood image of smoking is now out of date. I will stop smoking now because I am a modern man who is a health-conscious person.
- ❖ I know what I want and how to get it.
- ❖ I am a sociable man and a non-smoker

2.9 Action Plan 2: Act with Positive belief and, Show this in Attitudes about Smoking
- ❖ I believe that smoking is no longer a desirable habit.
- ❖ I will stop smoking now because I care about my health.

- ❖ I take particular care about my appearance because I like to feel good and look good, always.
- ❖ I will accomplish my goal by my decision and determination to stop smoking now!
- ❖ I accept that smoking is dangerous to my health and, I have made a firm decision to stop smoking because I am concerned to regain and improve my strength which has been weakened and my energy which has been dissipated by smoking.

2.10 Action Plan 3: Translating Action 2 into Positive Practical Action

- ❖ I care very much about eliminating smoke odour from my clothes and my body.
- ❖ I will always pay attention to my clothes and my personal hygiene.
- ❖ I will always pay attention to my overall appearance
- ❖ I will stop smoking completely and I will do so easily and effortlessly.
- ❖ I will refrain more and more from the habit of binge drinking of beer and wine.
- ❖ I will pay more attention to my overall physical appearance by doing exercises.
- ❖ I will practise the relaxation exercises outlined in this book.
- ❖ I will perform positive actions to stop smoking completely, easily, and effectively.

2.11 Action Plan 4: Be Confident in the Knowledge that You Are now a non-smoker

Knowing something entails knowing that one knows it. The *60 Cigarettes a Day Smoker* must profit from the knowledge that he or she is now a non-smoker. The benefit of this knowledge is that there are lapses such as falling prey to temptations in groups or gatherings where people smoke in order to belong. The worth of knowledge is in its usage. The *60 Cigarettes a Day Smoker* must make use of his newly acquired knowledge and show constantly that he is now a genuine non-smoker. He must accept himself as a non-smoker and, henceforth, regard smoking as a bad habit which is an anti-social habit.

* The *60 Cigarettes a day Smoker* must affirm the knowledge and belief which is expressed in action plans 1 and 2 by showing confidence in his ability to stop smoking now!
* The *60 Cigarettes a Day Smoker* must be positive about his decision and determination to stop smoking by making certain that this is reflected in his social behaviour and health concerns.
* The *60 Cigarettes a Day Smoker* must endeavour to make use of the knowledge that he is now a non-smoker and make the commitment to remain a non-smoker from this moment onwards.
* The *60 Cigarettes a day Smoker* must perform all the activities which are amenable to the fulfilment of the goal to stop smoking now.

2.12 Action Plan 5: Affirm the Goal

* The *60 Cigarettes a Day Smoker* must keep the goal constantly in his mind through a general positive outlook on the possibility of its attainment.
* The *60 Cigarettes a day Smoker* must **go for it** and stop smoking now completely, easily, effectively, and effortlessly in order to avoid the threat of bronchitis and emphysema, to feel good, look good and stop coughing.
* The *60 Cigarettes a Day Smoker* must affirm all the critical health and social reasons that were necessary for his journey to the world of positive possibilities (see chapter one). He must make that journey as often as necessary to maintain his non-smoker status.
* The general rule is for the *60 Cigarettes a Day Smoker* to remember his self worth and think of himself as a very sociable man who is a non-smoker (see action 1).

In the name of honesty, sincerity, and his concern for his health, the *60 Cigarettes a Day Smoker* must make a firm decision about his concern for his health if he is genuine and serious enough to stop smoking.

He must deal with conflict mentioned above by following the action plan rigidly in order to achieve the desired objective.

Notice that we have set the goal with a time element, *'Now!'* This time element is also part of the title of this book. It underlines both the urgency of the task in hand and the desire to stop smoking. It is the time element that transforms the *60 Cigarettes a Day Smoker's* desire to stop smoking now into a goal to stop smoking to look good and feel fit and healthy again.

The time element fixes the goal on the smoker's unconscious mind. The actions necessary to accomplish the goal have an additional effect of helping the smoker to stop smoking. The time element helps the smoker to be serious about the actions necessary to accomplish the goal and enables the smoker to keep the goal constantly in mind.

Notice also that the goal and the plans for its achievement involve the *60 Cigarettes a Day Smoker* in new activities and in positive thoughts which bring about positive feelings. I have used a gentleman's complaint for my illustration here. However, depending on the context of a problem, the same procedures are also applicable for a woman.

2.13 How to Acquire the Will to Succeed in Giving up Smoking
Remember that you must keep the goal alive to fulfil it. Refer to the fundamental principles of the mind technique in chapter one. You will find that the more deeply you understand the importance of the above factors, the more effectively you will be able to apply them in your daily life. In this way, you will be successful in whatever undertaking you embark on. You will certainly be successful in your goal to stop smoking completely, easily, effectively, and effortlessly. If you put your mind seriously into achieving success in your goal to stop smoking completely, easily, and effectively you must go for it so that you stop smoking now!

Use your mind positively. Give up all restrictive negative attitudes and propel yourself to success. Remember that in the quest for success in any endeavour, the success begins with a fellow's will to succeed. In every endeavour that you embark on, negative thoughts are the things that are most likely to prevent you from achieving the success that you desire. So, you must always avoid the temptation to engage in negatives thoughts in relation to your chosen goal.

Most important of all, you must always bear in mind the fundamental principles of the mind power technique which I have discussed in the first chapter of this book. Remember that the thought bricks for success or failure are constructed in the mind and always endeavour to construct the bricks for success. Try to understand and master the following little verse which clearly underlines the significance of the fundamental principles of the mind power technique which I discussed in chapter one of this book.

If you think you are beaten, you are.
If you think you dare not, you don't.
If you like to win, but think you can't,
It is a cinch you won't win.

If you think you will lose, you have lost.
For out of the world we find,
Success begins with a fellow's will,
It is all in the state of mind.
If you think you are outclassed, you are.
You've got to think high to rise,

You've got to be sure of yourself before
You can ever win a prize.
Life's battles don't always go
To the stronger or faster man,
But soon or late the man who wins
Is the man who thinks he can.
(Anonymous)

In any situation, if you think you can, you are already on your way to the winning post. It is all in the state of the mind. Your success begins with your construction of effective thought bricks which entails the plan of action which you have made to attain the success which you need. This is the essence of the power of the mind. Thus, you must always attune your mind to success and you will be for ever successful.

Remember that *the magic of success is within you.* It is within your mind. Apply the magic now in everything that you do from day to day starting from today and you will find that you can stop smoking now! You can do so completely, easily, and effectively by adhering to all the principles in this book.

CHAPTER THREE: STOP SMOKING COMPLETELY, EASILY, AND EFFECTIVELY

If you have built castles in the air, your work need not be lost: that is where they should be. Now put the foundations under them (Henry David Thoreau, 1817 - 1867).

3.1 Deep Relaxation as Weapon to Stop Smoking

I have discussed deep relaxation for the goal of giving up smoking in the last chapter. In this chapter, I offer you other ways of arriving at deep relaxation for the same purpose. Now you have a choice of what methods to adopt. The procedure, that is the outline of what to do, is the same but the scripts, imagery and pictorial representations are different.

Always remember that deep relaxation is an indispensable exercise to help you to stop smoking through our practical mind technique as it helps the individual to stay focused on the chosen objectives. To stop smoking completely, easily and effectively one must, first, learn how to attain a profound level of relaxation both mentally and physically. With practice, you will be able to attain your own required level of deep relaxation within minutes or seconds of your trying. It is that simple and I am going to show you how to try it right now. As the saying goes, *the taste of the pudding is in the eating*.

Most things within the field of depth psychology bear truth to the above saying. One can understand the techniques in the practice of depth psychology much better after one has experienced it through therapeutic analysis for self-knowledge, in the sense of finding out more about one's inner self. In like manner, in the case of mental exercises to stop smoking, one can focus much deeper on the chosen objective when one is deeply relaxed or when one has developed a relaxed attitude as a way of life.

I am dealing here with very practical personal affairs and the best method of approach in the application of practical matters is to practise by using the method that one wants to understand or learn about. With depth psychology, one does not need to be ill or emotionally unbalanced to learn to understand one's inner self. Before the experience of self knowledge some people are usually ignorant objectors, and a few may be uncritical apologists.

3.2 Practice Sessions

To practice how to focus the mind on the major goal to stop smoking completely, easily, and effectively, the individual must proceed with a method of deep relaxation as follows.

1. *Breathing Exercise*

Firstly, find a comfortable position either sitting on a chair or lying on a couch or on a bed, or on the floor if that is more comfortable for you. Now take a long, slow deep breath through your diaphragm. Hold your breath for a mental count of about 10, 20, 30, etc as desired. Choose the length of hold to suit your desired level of relaxation.

Then gently open your mouth slightly and slowly exhale as you allow the air out of your body and let go all negative thoughts as the air leaves your body and let go, let go, let go, let go, let go as you drift deeper, deeper, and deeper, into peace, allowing the feeling of relaxation to spread from the top of your head all the way down to your toes. Repeat the process three times.

This means that you will be performing four breathing exercises in all. If you have done this properly, as you read these lines, you should feel the sensation of relaxation moving through your body, now. Your body should now feel all loosened up.

However, if you do not feel loosened up at this stage it is because you are tense, nervous or fighting with yourself in being sceptical, doubting your own ability to do it well. If this is the case, do not worry. I tell you that you can do it; it is really very simple. Now let go your negative thoughts and negative feelings and repeat the procedure until you feel loosened up. Start now.

There is no fixed rule on how many times you can repeat the procedure. Many people feel at ease after one deep breathing exercise and some other people need to repeat the exercise a few times or several times to feel at ease. Do what suits you the best but, do the exercise. Do not skip it over because it is a necessary part of the deep relaxation in the practice of the method to stop smoking with the practical mind technique.

Remember the fundamental principles of the technical mind technique that I mentioned in chapter one. Try to think more about the great power of your mind and your ability to succeed in what you aim to achieve. If you truly believe that you can do it, you will. Always read the verse at the end of chapter two to encourage you and give you a confidence boost. However, if you feel any discomfort while doing the exercises, you must discontinue immediately and wait until you feel comfortable enough to continue.

2. Relaxation Exercise

When you have completed the breathing exercises, your next move is to relax every part of your body by focusing your thought or concentrating your attention on each part of your body that you wish to relax.

When you have mastered this technique of deep relaxation, you will find that at any time you direct your thoughts to any part of your body and say to that part (or command it) to *r e l a x,* it will immediately obey your command. It will begin to relax and you will start to feel at ease straight away. This may sound implausible to you at first but with practice you will be able to prove it for yourself. When this happens, you will be in control at any moment of tension or crisis.

In practising the techniques to stop smoking, you will be speaking directly to your unconscious mind. Since I have already discussed the power of the unconscious mind and how it records the data of your life, you can now see how you can stop smoking easily, completely and effectively. You can profit from your knowledge by recording your goals about stop smoking directly in your unconscious mind as I showed you in the last chapter.

This is part of the mental exercises which I mentioned above. It is an interesting exercise in this book. You will be programming your mind to do what you want, in this case, to effect deep relaxation in your life. In this way, you will be able to relax easily but, overall, the action plans for your goal will be manifested in your motor activity as you begin to perform, easily, effortlessly, all the everyday actions that are necessary to make your desire to stop smoking become a reality for you.

Note that it is much more effective to speak directly to your unconscious mind in the first person. However, you may speak in the second person if you prefer. This is effective too. If this is what you want, you can adapt the text here to speak in the second person. You can now begin to speak to your unconscious mind by telling it to effect deep relaxation in your body. You may begin with the relaxation process in the following way.

I am now entering a state of deep relaxation. My feet are becoming more and more deeply relaxed. This feeling of relaxation is spreading upwards from the tips of my toes through my feet to my ankles, legs, knees, and thighs. My limbs are getting more and more relaxed.

The feeling of relaxation increases from my thighs and spreads to my bottom, my waist, and my pelvis. This feeling of deep relaxation is slowly spreading to my abdomen, my stomach, my chest, and my back. I am getting more and more progressively relaxed. My entire body is becoming relaxed and I feel very light and, peaceful with relaxation.

Now, I shift my attention to my hands as this feeling of serenity is spreading to all parts of my body. My hands are becoming very deeply relaxed. The feeling of serenity and deep relaxation continues to flow upwards through my body from the tips of my fingers through my wrists, my hands, my elbows, my arms, all the way up to my shoulders.

Now as I am feeling relaxed, this feeling of relaxation surges across my shoulders so that my shoulders are deeply relaxed, very deeply relaxed. I now feel peace and tranquillity flowing through my whole body from all directions.

The feeling of relaxation continues to surge from my shoulders upwards to my neck and throat, and then across my face and up to the top of my head. My scalp, my forehead, my cheeks, and my jaw are all very deeply relaxed. I am now experiencing a very profound feeling of relaxation in every part of my body. Every consciousness and every system of my entire body is very deeply relaxed.

The whole of my body is now very deeply relaxed, peaceful and comfortable. My mind is calm, very quiet and tranquil. I am now perfectly in tune to give further information about giving up smoking to my unconscious mind. The information which I give will become part of my motor activity from now onwards and it will help me to give up smoking easily, completely and effectively.

Note that steps 1 and 2 above are known as *Induction*. In my discussion in the previous chapter, I have described this as *inducing yourself into a state of Deep Relaxation*. It is the same procedure but different way of arriving at deep relaxation. Do what suits you best.

3. The Instruction

You have now arrived at the crucial point at which to give dynamic instructions or mental prompts to your unconscious mind for your unconscious mind to produce the desired effect for you from now onwards. In the next section, I shall deal with how to give this information to your unconscious mind.

Basically, what I am saying is that when you have completed the breathing and the relaxation exercises correctly, you should be in the ideal frame of mind and disposition to programme your unconscious mind to effect the changes which you require in your life at any moment. In this instance, you need to speak to the unconscious mind about your desire to stop smoking easily, completely, and effectively.

Always remember the fundamental principles of the mind technique which I discussed in chapter one of this book. The thoughts that you have most often in your mind will become your reality. If the unconscious mind is fed constantly with your determination to stop smoking, this will become your reality and you will stop smoking easily, completely, effortlessly.

In this way, smoking will cease to feature in your consciousness because you will eliminate its effect by eliminating it from your life permanently. When you eliminate smoking from your life, you will do it easily, naturally, effortlessly, because your unconscious mind has got the message.

It is that simple but you need to be serious about it for this to happen. You need to be specific about your intentions and speak to the unconscious mind in unambiguous terms. Remember that the unconscious mind reproduces things exactly as you have presented them, just like a tape recorder. It is also important that you believe, wholly and firmly, in what you are saying to the unconscious mind and not merely verbalise it parrot fashion. Remember, also, that if you talk about doubts, doubt will become your reality and you will end up with uncertainty.

3.3 The Dynamics of Mental Prompts

Mental prompts are personal instructions or personal information which you give to your mind with the desire for the instruction or information to become your reality. The practical mind technique which I present to you in this book gives you the simplest method of recording information in the unconscious mind.

Remember that anything recorded in this way remains in the depth of unconsciousness but, it is at the same time very active as it affects an individual's motor actions. Everything that you say to the unconscious mind in a deep state of relaxation remains in the unconscious but is manifested in your everyday motor actions. If you have forgotten about the psychodynamics of the unconscious, you may now refer to my description of how the mind works in chapter 1.4.

Since your aim in reading this book is to stop smoking easily, completely and effectively, the information which you give to the unconscious mind will reflect this aim in order to make your desired status of non-smoker a reality. This method of recording information in the unconscious consists of personal instructions given by you to your unconscious mind thus facilitating instant replay of the required information in your everyday motor actions.

You will start in a simple way by giving simple information or instructions to the unconscious mind. Initially this will serve the purpose of getting yourself into the routine of giving mental prompts to the unconscious mind for the things which you desire to surface in your life through your everyday actions.

As you become adept in the use of mental prompts, you will find that the sky is the limit for you, because you can use the prompts to achieve anything you wish to achieve, to deal with anything in which you seek to achieve success. Indeed, to get what you want.

As you become relaxed and focus your mind deeply on what you wish to achieve, you will speak to your unconscious mind seriously about what you want to achieve. Soon with your actions, you will find that what you desire becomes your reality. Deep relaxation is the key to the success of mental prompts.

The personal instruction, or personal information, which I call mental prompts are mental directives ordering your unconscious mind to act on the information or instruction which you have given. Your unconscious mind acts on it to make your desire a reality. It works through your motor activities because, as I mentioned in chapter one and variously above, your unconscious mind acts on any information it receives.

Thus, the personal instructions, or personal information which you give to your unconscious mind must be direct, definite, simple and, preferably, given mentally. However, you may give your orders or instructions audibly if this is more convenient for you. You may choose to give your mental prompts in the way that is appropriate for you. However, you must take note that it must be given during the moment of ultimate deep relaxation as I mentioned above.

At this point of deepest relaxation, you have established the optimum conditions to give your mental prompts of personal instructions or personal information for your unconscious mind to receive them freely. This point of ultimate deep relaxation is the moment at which your mind is absolutely in receptive mode. You can see from this why it is more advisable to give the personal instructions or personal information mentally.

Whatever it is that you wish to accomplish in your life you can do so with the practical mind technique in this book. To use the technique, you will always make use of mental prompts but as I have mentioned above, it is always best to use the mental prompts technique of personal information or personal instruction immediately during the moment of ultimate deep relaxation.

If you have a lot of different instructions or information to give to your mind, you will find that it is very beneficial to put these in a sequence that is logical and meaningful to you. Remember that your unconscious mind is uncritical. It does not change your instructions, it merely reproduces what you say, faithfully, to you. Thus, you must take care in the knowledge that your unconscious mind accepts information as presented. If what you say is careless, meaningless, or ambiguous, your desired reality will not materialise as you want it, or it may not materialize at all!

It is also important that your mental prompts which consist of the personal instructions or personal information that you give to your unconscious mind should be in your own words, words that, as mentioned above, are meaningful to you and tailored to each specific area, problem, or situation in your life which you wish to confront. Do not be rigid about this. Do whatever suits your requirements and what works best for you.

Give your instructions or personal information and, then relax and allow the unconscious mind to work on your instructions to make the instructions effective for you. For example, after you have used the relaxation technique and you feel that you are in the moment of ultimate deep relaxation, you may let your first personal instruction be to direct your unconscious mind to accept the word *r e l a x* as your instant cue for deep relaxation. You may begin to give this direction as follows.

From this moment onwards, wherever I happen to be, whatever the occasion, whatever the circumstances, whomever I happen to be with, when I use the word 'r e l a x', I will become deeply relaxed immediately, comfortable and serene as I am now. The word 'r e l a x' will mean complete calm, peace, and total deep relaxation in my entire being.

This is an excellent positive instruction at this stage because by it you are instructing your unconscious mind to make the feeling of deep relaxation a part of your life. What will happen with this mental prompt is that the feeling of deep relaxation will become an attitude of mind and body for you and you will cease to feel tense, edgy, nervous, or irritable. You will be relaxed in difficult situations, come what may, you will be in control, calm, relaxed in mind and body.

Notice that in the above instruction I said that *"I will become deeply relaxed immediately, comfortable and serene as I am now"*. This is because the instructions should be given during the moment in your relaxation exercise when you attain a state of ultimate deep relaxation and feel peaceful and serene.

The purpose of the instruction, therefore, is to allow your unconscious mind to save this moment for you and make it a permanent part of your life which you can playback or bring on at any time you use the word *r e l a x*. Remember this, always. The essence of this is that you can order it at any time and receive it because it is already there for you.

This act of giving simple instruction to your unconscious mind will bring about positive results in your life in whatever goal you wish to accomplish. It is important to distinguish the act of ordering, commanding, or giving instructions to your mind from the act of giving suggestions.

The act of ordering, commanding, or giving instructions to your unconscious mind involves you in making a positive demand from your unconscious mind, ordering it to do what you want. It is like placing an order for something. Remember also the powerful force of the positive instructions in the preparatory exercise at the beginning of chapter one.

In the above example, you are giving an order which is to be executed by your unconscious mind to the extent that each time you use the word *r e l a x,* you will feel, from that moment onwards, an automatic and instant deep relaxation in mind and body.

Your command will also bring about a highly desirable state of total calm whenever you desire it and wherever you happen to be, whether you are travelling on a crowded train, taking an examination, having a job interview, in a business meeting, participating in competitive sports event, driving a car in a busy traffic or in moments of minor personal crisis.

All you need to do in the situations above is to say the word *r e l a x* and you will feel deeply relaxed, instantly.

The same procedure applies in giving up smoking. Remember that it is necessary to be specific when making mental prompts. You must be clear and specific about the fact that you wish to give up smoking easily, completely, and effectively. This is what you will ask for in your universal mental prompt or mind order. You want to eliminate smoking from your consciousness and become a non-smoker. This is what you will ask for or order for in your mental prompts.

3.4 Exercises to Stop Smoking
Here I present further relaxation exercises which will help you to stop smoking easily, completely, effectively, and effortlessly. You do not need to use all of them at the same time although you may go through them and settle on the one that makes you feel comfortable. Remember that each of the exercises to stop smoking in the previous chapters and the ones that I present in this section begins with a method for deep relaxation. Follow the procedure which is given above. This procedure is incorporated in the exercises given below.

Using Deep Relaxation as a method for Induction
Settle down on a comfortable chair, bed, or on the floor. Close your eyes and feel yourself relaxing gently as you keep your eyes firmly closed. Now imagine or picture, if you can, a scene of peace and tranquillity like the gushing of waves on a sandy shore, leaves rustling in a gentle breeze or whatever scene represents peace and tranquillity to you. Remember that the thoughts, pictures, and images you have in your mind constantly are the things that will materialise into reality for you as these are charged with energy.

Now take a long, slow, deep breath through your diaphragm. Hold the breath to a count of 5, or 10, or whatever number that is appropriate for you. Now open your mouth gently and breathe out slowly as you feel yourself, going deeper, and deeper, and deeper into relaxation becoming more and more progressively relaxed with each breath that you take and with each moment.

Now take a second long, slow deep breath through your diaphragm. Hold the breath to a count of 5, 10, or the number that is appropriate to you, as before. Open your mouth gently and breathe out slowly as you let the air out of your body and relax, relax, going deeper and deeper, and deeper with each breath and with each moment.

Now take a third long, slow, deep breath through your diaphragm and hold to a count of 5, or 10, as you wish as before. Now open your mouth and this time as you let the air out of your body gently, I want you to count the numbers from 10 to zero and relax as you go deeper, deeper, deeper, and deeper into relaxation.

Using the Vibrant Energy of the Sun to Bring Peace and Serenity
Since I am appealing here to the benefits of the vibrant energy of the light of the sun, it is best to use this exercise during the day time. If you have an urgent need to use it during the night time, you must modify the text to suit your purpose. Otherwise, use one of the other exercises in the previous chapters or the ones that I give below.

Those people who are not comfortable with the light of the sun can also use one of the other exercises given below, as I have provided a choice of exercises for everyone. You can also use the exercises interchangeably if you prefer.

Now that you have completed the breathing exercise, I will use the vibrant energy of the light of the sun to relax every part of your body. The light of the sun can be your instant cue to deep relaxation so that whenever you reach out, mentally, and bring the light of the sun over to your body you will feel deeply relaxed instantly.

The light of the sun is, truly, your light in the dark. It helps you to see your way clearly wherever you are going, and it signposts the directions for you. The light of the sun guides you in whatever you are doing.

The light of the sun is a positive light. It helps you to achieve positive results with your goals, wishes and desires.

Here, I have written everything for you, in the first person. You can change the text if you feel more comfortable to give your instructions in the second person. It is effective, too.

Now, I see myself out in the open air on a beautiful day. At this moment, I can choose to be in a park on a beach or on a holiday. The important thing is that wherever it is that I have chosen to be in my mind is a place which represents for me the very ultimate in peace, joy, and total relaxation.

I believe that the light of the sun is a healing light, a positive light, a light that represents joy, happiness, total fulfilment, and every positive thing which I wish to feature in my life. The successful achievement of my goal is represented by the warmth of the healing rays of the light of the sun around me.

The light of the sun symbolises my success, my joy, my happiness, and my achievement of my goal to stop smoking and fulfil my wish. Whenever I bring the light of the sun into my life, I feel good instantly because it energises me. It helps me to think positive thoughts about myself and the fulfilment of my goal. The light of the sun is a magical light because it brings success to me instantly, effortlessly. The light of the sun is my cue to instant deep relaxation in mind and body. Whenever I bring the light of the sun over to my body, I feel deeply relaxed, instantly.

It is a beautiful day today. The light from the sun is warm and shining down through my body and it makes me feel good, positive, and deeply relaxed. I want to stay with this feeling and I notice now that the sky is an incredibly beautiful blue and there is a comforting breeze blowing across my body. I feel peaceful and deeply relaxed.

Now, I am reaching up to bring the light of the sun to my body. I bring it over to my right arm and focus it there like the ray or beam of a torch light and I move it from the tips of my fingers, through the palm of my hand, my wrists, my lower arm, my elbow, my upper arm, all the way up to my shoulders.

I move the light of the sun backwards and forward, up, and down until I can feel it in my mind as the warmth of the light of the sun penetrates my skin, my muscles, my nerves and the bones in my body. I can feel my entire body beginning to relax more and more, deeper, and deeper, I am becoming more deeply relaxed every minute.

Now I move the light of the sun from my right arm to my left arm and from the tips of my fingers upwards through my wrist, my lower arm, my elbow, my upper arm, to my shoulders. I move the light of the sun backwards and forward and I can feel my left arm going deeply relaxed as my entire body settles down into deep relaxation and my sense and feeling of peace and tranquillity increases.

Now, I shift my attention and bring the light of the sun over to my right leg and I move it from the tips of my toes through my feet, my ankle, my lower leg, my knee, my upper leg, all the way up to my hip. As I breathe gently, I can feel my muscles relaxing and I can concentrate more and more on thinking positive thoughts about my goals. My right leg and my toes all the way to my hip go deeply relaxed, very deeply relaxed.

Now I move the light of the sun from my right leg to my left leg and from my toes through my feet, my ankle, my lower leg, my knee, my upper leg, all the way to my hip and I feel my left leg relaxing deeper and deeper and deeper.

Now with both of my legs very, very deeply relaxed and both of my arms very deeply relaxed, I am using my own breathing as my guide to total relaxation and I can feel my entire body going deeper and deeper into relaxation with each breath that I take and, with each positive thought and positive feeling that I have, with each moment, I am becoming increasingly deeply relaxed.

The author tells me that some people feel light and weightless when they are deeply relaxed; that they feel as weightless as if they could just float away. He says that other people experience a tingling sensation all over their body when they are deeply relaxed while some others have a feeling of elation or a feeling of peace and contentment.

Now, I firmly believe that whatever feeling I have at this moment should be a positive feeling which is right and proper for me in relation to my goal. I want to stay with my positive feeling and allow my mind to settle down as I go deeper, deeper, and deeper into relaxation.

Now, I bring the light from the sun gently into my stomach and I feel it beginning to warm and to glow over my stomach. I feel it glowing like a ball of vibrant energy and I feel the energy in every organ in my body. I can respond positively to this healing energy from the light of the sun as every organ in my body relaxes and I feel peaceful.

I can feel the newfound peace and tranquillity in my life as each day brings joy and contentment to me and my mind is filled with new and positive things to do which in their turn, make me feel peaceful, confident, and optimistic about myself and about the future. I want to stay with my peaceful feeling as I go deeper, deeper, and deeper into relaxation.

Now, as I move the light of the sun into my heart and my chest I can experience, feel, and know what it feels like to take this healing energy of the sun into my body, into my blood stream. I can feel it as it moves out into every organ in my body and every organ is responding, healing and relaxing. I notice now that my mind is becoming very peaceful and I have a feeling of joy and happiness. This is how things will be for me from now onwards.

Now, I shift my attention to my back. I bring the light of the sun to my back and I move it gently up and down my back. I move it across your back. I feel it massaging my back as the feeling of relaxation spreads from my upper back to my lower back and across my waist as the whole of my back goes deeply relaxed, very deeply relaxed.

Now as I bring the light of the sun into my body through my head automatically my brain guides the light through my spinal cord to the tip of my spine. I notice that when the light gets to the tip of my spine, it begins to move out to all areas of my body. From the tip of my spine, the light begins to radiate to every part of my body and every part of my body is relaxing accordingly.

I can feel it now as the healing light of the sun is radiating to every organ in my body and every organ in my body is becoming active, alive, and relaxing deeply. Every organ in my body is becoming healed by the light of the sun and every organ is now functioning and harmonising as it should. I will continue to relax more and more and allow the healing process to begin in my body. I will allow the positive changes to take place in my body and in my life from now onwards.

Now as the light from the sun moves across my shoulders, I feel very much at ease. As I move the light of the sun from my shoulders, through my neck and my throat, I notice that my forehead relaxes, my scalp relaxes, my neck and my throat relax, the muscles around my eyes and cheeks relax. Now, I will allow every part of my face to relax freely and allow myself to go into a deeper, more blissful, more comfortable state of relaxation.

I am now relaxed, very deeply relaxed. I am at ease with what is happening now in my mind and body and very much at peace with what is being made available to me now.

In a few moments, I will be giving mental prompts to my unconscious mind asking it to receive certain information or instructions from me and to act on it as part of my everyday motor activities. These mental prompts will act to strengthen my determination to stop smoking, my desire, my will power and my self-control. The mental prompts will fortify me in mind and body and will make it possible for me to maintain my integrity and my goal to stop smoking. I believe that each mental prompt that I give to my unconscious mind will have a unique effect upon me.

The mental prompts will grow stronger and stronger in me and become more and more effective for me from this moment onwards. The mental prompts will become totally a complete part of my everyday motor behaviour, totally and completely effective for me immediately.

I can also add to the strength and effectiveness of the mental prompts because from now onwards, each time I have a longing or a great desire to smoke I will be automatically reminded to count the numbers down mentally from ten to zero and, as I do this, I will notice that my longing or desire to smoke is easily eliminated.

Each time I do this I will find that the mental prompts have a unique effect on me. I will always remember the essential principle that the ideas which I have most often in my mind will become my reality. I will always remember the power of the unconscious mind in relation to mental prompts.

I am now very deeply relaxed, very, very deeply relaxed. I feel a definite sense of peace moving over my body. Now I imagine myself back on that beautiful place in the open air where I was a moment ago. I will be there at the count of five to zero. Five, four, three, two, one, zero. I am there.

I notice that the light from the sun is warm and shining down around my body and I have a feeling of peace, tranquillity, and total relaxation. As I continue to relax in this way, I will find that through the days and nights from now onwards, with my positive thoughts and my desire to stop smoking, and my increased deep relaxation, the thoughts and desires of smoking have been eliminated easily and effortlessly.

Each mental prompt that I give here will be a permanent part of me for my mind is being programmed now to receive the mental prompts and I will act on them automatically, involuntarily, unconsciously. I will begin carrying out the dictates of the mental prompts in my motor activities and they will become effective for me immediately. These mental prompts will change my attitude to smoking because I now have much more self control, much more will power and much more determination to succeed in my desire to stop smoking than ever before.

Now, I want to stay relaxed and go deeper, deeper, and deeper. I want to realise from now onwards that with each passing day I have the power to obtain whatever I desire. The power to get whatever I desire is truly within me and my desire at this moment is so intense that I can now visualize myself as a non-smoker because that is what I desire. I will always remember my mental journey to the new world of positive possibilities. I can make that journey again at any time I choose as it will help me to actualize my goal to stop smoking and any other goal that I might have.

Cleaning and Purifying your Lungs

Now that I am deeply relaxed, I want to make an investigative journey into the inside of my body. I want to see what it is like in relation to my smoking habit. I will get there at a count of five to zero. Five, four, three, two, one, zero. I am now inside my own body. I notice, immediately, that the inside of my body needs cleaning and, that there is an anti-bacterial liquid detergent inside my body. This liquid will clean, disinfect, and purify my internal system. The liquid has two vital roles to fulfil for me in relation to my wish to stop smoking.

The first vital role of the liquid is that as a detergent, it will purge all my desire and thoughts of smoking and wash these out of my mind and out of my internal system for good. The second vital role of the liquid is its cleansing work in my lungs. The liquid will wipe out the deposits of tar, nicotine and the poisons from my lungs and keep my lungs and my internal system fresh. This will enable me to have clean lungs and regular fresh breath. It will, also, enhance my desire to live a healthy life style from now onwards.

Now, I want to concentrate my attention on my lungs. I listen, quietly, to the cleaning work that is being down by the anti-bacterial liquid. I can feel it now, scrubbing, cleaning my lungs. It feels good, it is a pleasant sensation but, I notice that there is still more work of cleaning to be done.

Now I want to step in and take control regarding the health of my lungs and my health in general. So, now, I imagine that I am a cleaner inside my lungs. My job is to go into my lungs and clean it out thoroughly. I will be there at the count of five to zero. Five, four, three, two, one, zero. I am now a cleaner in my lungs.

Now, I notice that my lungs are as dark as the inside of a chimney and there is a mass of wreckage, soot and rubbish left there by the effect of smoke. My job is to clear the mass of rubbish and to clean my lungs of the tar, the nicotine and the poisons that are left there by the impact of smoke. I can use whatever is necessary and I can use the liquid detergent to help me. I will begin the cleaning work now.

Now I clean both sides of my lungs. I clean them up and down. I clean out all the filthy rubbish and I use the liquid antibacterial detergent to make my lungs fresh and free from odour. My cleaning work will leave my lungs feeling fresh. In this way I will always have fresh breath. My work is done. I believe that I have done an excellent job.

Now, my next job is to move from my lungs to my spine. I want to get there at the count of five to zero. Five, four, three, two, one, zero. I am now in my spine. Here, I notice that many of the nerves of my body are connected to my spine and the nerves have been severely damaged and ravaged by the effects of smoking.

My job now is to take the sponge that is in the liquid detergent and use it to apply the liquid gently on my nerves from my spine all the way to my brain. I notice, as I apply the liquid to my nerves, that my nerves are becoming relaxed and the ravages and damage in them are healed. I continue to do this from my spine to the centre of my brain in an engine room where all the sockets and plugs with smoking are connected. From here, I begin now to apply the liquid to my nerves to repair the damage caused by the effect of smoke.

Pulling out the Plugs and Sockets from unnecessary Smoking Connections
I have applied the liquid to my nerves from my spine to my brain and I am now in an engine room at the centre of my brain. Now, I look around the engine room and I notice that the engine room is the electrical power station of my brain, with many plugs and sockets connected.

These plugs, sockets and their connections represent my emotional, mental, physical and psychological association with the unwanted habit of smoking. My job now is to disconnect the plugs and sockets. As I disconnect them, I will disconnect myself now and permanently from the unwanted habit of smoking and I will stop smoking for good.

Now, I notice that there is a plug and socket for every association with smoking. There is a plug which represents my first smoke of the day. Now, I will reach out in my mind and discount the plug and socket which represent my first smoke of the day. This will help me to stop smoking now.

I used to associate smoking with the feeling of relaxation but I realized right now that I am very deeply relaxed now without smoking and that I can be relaxed easily, completely, effectively, and peacefully at any time I choose, without smoking. So, I disconnect the plug and socket that associates smoking with a feeling of relaxation. This will help me to stop smoking now.

I will pull out the plug and socket that connects with my habit of smoking before eating, during eating, or after eating a meal and I will stop smoking. From now onwards I will enjoy perfect health with increased stamina and vitality because I am eating without smoking before, during or after a meal.

In the past, I had associated smoking with being in control, being smart, being fashionable, being superior or being in authority. Now, I must pull the socket and plug that connects smoking to these situations, positions and attitudes and I will stop smoking immediately for I can be all these things more effectively, without smoking.

I had associated smoking with a fashionable, friendly and sociable activity which is performed on social occasions but, now, I must pull out the socket and plug which associates smoking with being fashionable, friendly, and sociable. I will stop smoking now because I realize now that it is quite alright for me to be friendly, fashionable, and sociable without smoking.

Some people turn to smoking as a solution to certain emotional problems in their lives or they may be insecure and turn to smoking for some superficial social reasons. I must now pull out the socket and plug which represent any attempt on my part to solve emotional problems by smoking. I must stop smoking immediately because smoking creates and aggravates emotional problems.

Some smokers use smoking as a form of oral gratification. They have an unfulfilled, unconscious, need to put something in their mouth as a substitute for what is lacking. I will cease to use smoking as a form of oral gratification and I must now pull out the socket and plug that represents any attempt on my part to use smoking as a substitute, oral gratification. I must pull out the socket and plug now to stop smoking immediately.

Some people have been badly influenced into smoking by the Hollywood image of famous film stars smoking. These people feel that smoking will make them appear mature, attractive, and sophisticated like the Hollywood stars that they idolize. I am now very aware that the idea which is conjured by the image of the big stars of Hollywood smoking is now out of date and unfashionable.

I must pull out the socket and plug that represent the image of Hollywood stars smoking because I know now that smoking is an antisocial habit which is no longer permitted in many public places. I will stop smoking now and embrace a new way of living with care and concern for my health and wellbeing.

There are other people who smoke because they suffer from peer pressure. For these people, smoking is the only way that they can belong with the peers. I am a free spirit who is positive, confident, optimistic, and very much in control of my private life. I am very secure in myself. So, I must pull out the socket and plug that associate smoking with peer pressure and being a member of a gang. I have stopped smoking now.

I have disconnected many of the sockets and plugs that represent various associations with smoking. Now, I notice that there is only one socket and plug left. This is the socket and plug that represent my last smoke of the day. Now, I will pull out the last socket and plug which represent my last smoke of the day and I will disconnect myself from smoking for ever. I will stop smoking immediately. I will pull out the socket and plug now! I believe that I have done an excellent work in disconnecting the bad habit of smoking from my life, permanently.

The cleansing of my internal system is now complete. The liquid detergent has done its job effectively and it is now time to allow what is left of it to flow out of my body. It will flow out of my body at the count of five to zero. Five, four, three, two, one, zero. I will allow the liquid detergent to flow out of my body now.

As the liquid detergent flows out of my body, it carries with it the very thought of smoking itself, the nicotine, tar and poisons. As the liquid flows out of my body, I can see how filthy and repulsive it is. As the liquid detergent now flows completely out of my body, I will have a look at my lungs now. I notice that my lungs now look clean and fresh and that I am now breathing clearer and easier.

I am now deeply relaxed, very, very deeply relaxed. I have a feeling of peace and total relaxation moving all over my body. Now, I imagine myself back in that place in the open air, on a beautiful day. I will be there at the count of five to zero. Five, four, three, two, one, zero. I am there now. I notice that the light of the sun is warm and shining down around my body. The atmosphere is beautiful with comforting breeze blowing across my body and the feeling is one of peace and contentment.

I have the knowledge that I have now given up smoking and I have done so easily, effectively, effortlessly.

I will now instruct my unconscious mind with powerful, positive, mental prompts which will be very beneficial to me. Each mental prompt will become part of my everyday motor response or motor behaviour. I will act on them automatically and they will become effectively immediately because they are powerfully constructed to help me to stop smoking now!

From now onwards, I will think positive thoughts so that positive feelings will flow to me, automatically, about my new status as a non-smoker. Whenever negative thoughts of smoking attempt to enter my mind and consciousness I must cancel them immediately by focusing my mind on my new status as a non-smoker. I will take a long, slow deep breath through my diaphragm and count the numbers from ten, nine, eight, seven, six, five, four, three, two, one, zero.

I will notice that each time I cancel negative thoughts from my mind, and take a long, slow, deep breath through my diaphragm and count the numbers down from ten to zero, I become more relaxed, positive, and resolute as a non-smoker. With practice this will become more effective for me as the very thought of smoking will be eliminated from my life permanently.

I have now stopped smoking. From now onwards I will become more and more relaxed with people, with members of my family and the people with whom I associate in daily life. Members of my family and my close associates will notice the change in my attitudes to smoking and how it has brought pleasant changes in me as a person and they will all be delighted for me and with what I have achieved. This will encourage me, even more, to stop smoking for ever.

From this moment onwards my impulse, desire, need, habit or urge for smoking has been terminated for ever. Smoking has now lost its hold on me as I now regard smoking as a sign of immaturity and insecurity.

I recognised that there is a great deal about smoking that is unpleasant so I made the great decision to stop smoking and, having stopped smoking, I will experience the most tremendous sense of accomplishment.

I am now a non-smoker and my determination, my self-control, my will power and my self-respect have all increased. I know now that smoking is a harmful and dangerous habit. I am now aware that smoking can lead to heart disease, lung cancer, emphysema, bronchitis, which may lead to bronchiectasis and bronchiolitis.

I am now aware that smoking has a dangerous effect on a person's sex life as it lowers the fertility rate in women and reduces sperm count in men. I am now aware of the amount of money involved in smoking and how I would love to use the money to do something beneficial for myself, for my family, or for the people around me.

I am aware of the dangers of smoking to children, unborn babies, and the people around me all of whom have been forced to become passive smokers by my selfish habit of smoking around them. I am now aware of the unhygienic effects of smoking such as the smell of smoke which I carry along with me, bad breath, ashes on my clothing, stained teeth, and stained fingers.

When I consider these problems, which are related to smoking, I make the wise decision to stop smoking immediately. From the moment that I stopped smoking I will begin to feel better during the day and I will begin to sleep more soundly at night, my health will improve and my mind will be clear and alert and I will feel better about life generally.

I will have much more self control, determination and will power to resist the temptation to smoke. I will be able to resist the temptation to overeat and so I will maintain my ideal weight because my mind controls what I eat.

Now that I have stopped smoking and smoking is now in my past, I am very glad that it is now over, that I have given up the bad habit of smoking and I have done so easily and effortlessly. I have now developed a special feeling of superiority over the people who smoke because I know that they lack my self-control, my determination, my will power, my sense of self-worth and self-respect. From now onwards, smoking will cease to feature in my consciousness. I have stopped smoking and I feel very good about myself and my wise decision to stop smoking.

Now, I will take a long, slow deep breath through my diaphragm and count the numbers down from ten to zero. I will be ten times more deeply relaxed and I will relax on each descending number. Every number down will be a step to peace and contentment and this will give me a feeling of accomplishment. I will count the numbers down, now. Ten, nine, eight, seven, six, five, four, three, two, one, zero.

Whenever I take a long, slow, deep breath through my diaphragm and count the numbers down from ten to zero, my determination, my will power, and my self-control will be strengthened making it easy for me to maintain my resolution to stop smoking now!

I will carry out all the positive mental prompts, or suggestions that my unconscious mind has accepted and recorded faithfully for me and these will become effective in my life. These positive mental prompts or suggestions will become stronger for me and they will grow stronger day by day in every way and I will be happy that I have stopped smoking for ever.

A Retrospective Journey
I am now going to move forward in time to allow me to look back in time and experience myself as a non-smoker who is thrilled by the joy and happiness of giving up smoking for ever. This journey forward in time is like my journey to the world of positive possibilities. At the end of the journey, I will return to the world of actuality to actualize everything. I must remember to acknowledge that as I am able to visualize it, I will, also, actualize it.

At the count of five to zero, I will imagine that it is now six months since I stopped smoking and I am feeling good about myself. Five, four, three, two, one, zero. It is now six months since I stopped smoking and I am feeling good about myself. I feel relaxed by such thoughts as I move forward and forward in time.

At the next count of five to zero, it will be one year since I stopped smoking and I am feeling terrific about my wise decision to stop smoking and about the general improvement in my health since I stopped smoking. Five, four, three, two, one, zero. It is now one year since I stopped smoking and I am feeling terrific. I am very deeply relaxed, as I move forward and forward in time.

At the next count of five to zero, it will be two years since I stopped smoking and I will be feeling happy that I have stopped the bad habit of smoking. The number now is five, four, three, two, one, zero. It is now two years since I stopped smoking and I am feeling quite happy about it. I am deeply relaxed, as I move forward and forward in time.

At the next count of five to zero, it will be three years since I stopped smoking and I will be feeling wonderful about myself. Five, four, three, two, one, zero. It is now three years since I stopped smoking and I am feeling absolutely, wonderful, day by day in every way. I will continue to be relaxed from day to day and relish my sense and feeling of accomplishment.

I am now relaxed, very, very deeply relaxed and I am happy knowing that I have made a positive decision to stop smoking and I have made the decision easily, firmly and correctly. My mind is continuously in the moment of now and I take credit for my success with each passing day in the knowledge that I have stopped smoking for ever.

Now, I want to bring the power of the healing light of the sun with its positive energy to energise me and maintain my status as a non-smoker. I bring it over to the top of my head to relax me and to cleanse me. Day by day in every way from now onwards, I will have much more energy and vitality as the effect of my positive decision to make changes in my life by giving up the bad habit of smoking. I will feel happy by this in the knowledge that I have stopped smoking for ever.

Now, as I count the numbers upwards from one to five, I will become alert to what I have achieved at the count of five. My mind will become clear and I will feel refreshed and alert, healthier and feeling much better than I have ever felt before. I will be able to go about my normal activities and face my day (or night) with renewed strength, energy, joy, happiness, and vitality with the knowledge that I have stopped smoking for ever.

1. I can feel the energy entering my body, moving into every part of my body. I am slowly getting ready to come up, now.
2. I am beginning now to move my hands and feet as I slowly come up. I am feeling incredibly alive and happy with a smile on my face.
3. I am now moving up slowly and stretching, feeling good, coming up, up, up, with the knowledge that I have now stopped smoking and I have done so easily and effortlessly.
4. There is a broad smile on my face, a warm, more comfortable feeling of accomplishment with the knowledge that from now onwards I will have more energy and vitality.
5. The number 5 has been counted. I can open my eyes now and sit up with a clear knowledge that I have stopped smoking and I have done so easily and effortlessly. I acknowledge, happily, that I have done well. I am now a non-smoker.

3.5 Positive Suggestions to Stop Smoking
An Alternative Method

In this exercise, you can use any of the techniques for deep relaxation and induction which I have given in the exercises in the previous sections and chapters. The chief aim in this exercise is to emphasise the positive aspect of being a non-smoker as I draw your attention to the detriments of being a smoker.

Basically, this exercise is intended to make the smoker to become averse to the habit of smoking. I give the instructions here in the second person but you can alter the text to the first person in the way that I have written for you in the previous examples.

Now I want you to cast your mind back to your journey to the new world of positive possibilities. I want you to reflect for a moment on the health and social reasons which made the journey a necessary journey for you.

As you reflect on this, you will find from now onwards that you will be more and more strongly aware of the reasons to stop smoking and you will be more and more conscious of the threat to your health, of the increased chance of dying an ugly, painful, death from heart disease or cancer. You will be aware of the threat of fighting for each breath with bronchitis or emphysema or of causing sever damage to the arteries or veins in your body.

Many hardened smokers try to dismiss these threats and comfort themselves with the thought that it takes a long time to die from smoking. It is true that people do not die directly from smoking but each puff from smoking is a direct contributory cause of smoking related diseases whose threat become imminent as you continue to smoke.

Even now you will notice the way smoking interferes with your healthy life style, the gradual decline in your health, fitness and stamina, the shortness of breath which you get when you try to run, play other sports, or climb stairs. There is also the bad breath that comes with smoking and the loss of the sense of smell and sense of taste.

You will ponder on the cost of smoking. Think about how much money you are spending on smoking from week to week, month to month or within one year. Work out this amount and think of how you could have used this amount to improve your health or to do something more beneficial to yourself or to members of your family.

From this moment onwards, you will be more and more aware that smoking is becoming less and less acceptable in public and in social places. Smoking is now an anti-social behaviour in public places because it is dangerous to the people around you and you are, callously, forcing them to become passive smokers against their will.

Some people smoke because they think that smoking makes them feel big, relaxed, and important but you know, deep down, that smoking makes smokers tense, nervous, snappy and irritable. Smoking is a nauseating habit. You will notice that if you continue to smoke from now onwards, you will be embarrassed and disgusted with yourself for being involved with such an anti-social and unhealthy habit and you will have an overwhelming unpleasant, sickening, feeling of nausea.

The unpleasant, dangerous, effects of smoking will take over in your mind and you will notice that you will no longer be able to smoke. When this happens, you will know that your urge to smoke has disappeared and that smoking has lost its hold on you.

In addition to your realization of the unpleasant, dangerous effects of smoking, your unconscious mind knows all your reasons for wishing to stop smoking and it will find a safe way for you to stop smoking now because the reasons for your necessary journey to the new world of positive possibilities are imprinted on your unconscious mind. This can be played back to you each time you reflect on the journey to the world of positive possibilities.

When this happens, you will be unable to smoke again for your desire to smoke will be dissolved by your unconscious mind and, your craving for any method of smoking will disappear completely from your life. From that moment onwards, smoking will be very repugnant to you and you will develop a feeling of superiority over the people who smoke because you know that you have acquired a new social behaviour as a non-smoker and that smokers are anti-social.

From the moment that you stopped smoking, you will cease to notice and acknowledge smokers because the habit of smoking has been dissolved from your life and it has gone out of your consciousness. You will feel confident, positive, and optimistic with the knowledge that you have stopped smoking for ever.

As your confidence grows with your new knowledge, you will become more and more proud of your self control, your self respect, your determination, and your will power. You will feel healthier and look healthier, you will breathe well, your lungs will be cleaner, you will have more energy and your level of fitness and stamina will be greatly increased. You will feel good about yourself and about your life and your new life style as you discover that you can enjoy life more beneficially without smoking.

You will be calm and very much relaxed day by day in every way. As you are now a non-smoker, you will notice that you enjoy your food better as it tastes better because the bad taste in your mouth and the bad breath associated with smoking are now gone and out of your life.

As you become more and more relaxed from day to day, you will begin to pay more attention to your health in general and you will be eating healthy food to remain healthy always. In view of your new healthy regime and healthy eating habits, you will see that you will be able to enjoy your food and maintain your ideal weight when it is necessary to do so.

You will, also, be able to protect your body from the dangerous effect of nicotine, tar and poisons which may come from the threat of further smoking.

As you continue to pay great attention to your health and enjoying healthy foods, you will feel stronger and stronger, healthier and healthier, from now onwards. In this way, your resistance to smoking related illness and disease will increase and become stronger, steadily, day by day in every way.

You know that for the sake of your health and social life, it makes very good sense to stop smoking. Your journey to the new world of positive possibilities has been beneficial to you enormously. It has helped you to realize the necessity to stop smoking and you have stopped smoking completely and permanently.

You have now stopped smoking completely, easily, and effectively. You have done so effortlessly with the power of your unconscious mind which records your positive intentions. Now you can count the numbers from one to five as in the previous exercises, to come out of deep relaxation, successfully. Well Done.

3.6 How to make the habit of Non-smoking Your Reality
You can stop smoking easily, effectively, and effortlessly because you have a firm desire to be a non-smoker. Your desire will become your

reality soon. Remember that the thoughts which you have most often in your mind become your reality. If you can bring your thoughts into pictures and see them clearly then you can realise them easily and effortlessly. This is one way in which your dreams become your reality.

In this relaxation exercise, you will learn how to picture your desires and realise them. Remember also the journey to the world of positive possibilities in the preparatory exercise in chapter one. You can make the same journey now and try to see yourself as a non-smoker so that this will become your reality in the actual world.

To perform this exercise effectively, follow the steps as in the previous relaxation exercises and concentrate on seeing yourself as a non-smoker. Visualize yourself as you would like to be and use effective mental prompts from the moment of your optimum relaxation.

3.7 Going for Your Success to Stop Smoking with Confidence

If you have followed everything that I have discussed here so far with attention then you have grasped the essential ingredients of the recipe for success in the use of your mind to get what you want. Always remember that whatever success you achieve in whatever field comes through your effective use of your mind to build an impregnable mind castle.

You must now consolidate on what you have gained from this book. To do this you must display confidence in yourself and in your ability to succeed in your chosen field, that is, in your ability to stop smoking now easily, completely, and effortlessly.

You can display this confidence by translating the secrets you have found in this book, your new pattern of belief system, your new wealth of ideas regarding the unpleasant and dangerous effects of smoking, your positive attitudes and positive frame of mind in respect to yourself and your goals and aspiration, etc, into action. Always be resolute and positive about your desire to achieve success with your stop smoking programme. I have discussed various mind techniques to stop smoking in this chapter and various methods of relaxation in this book.

Practise the method that you feel most comfortable with but you must practise because action is the essential ingredient that brings success in any goal. Action is the route to change. You are making changes in your life by your desire to stop smoking.

Now, you must take the bull by the horn with courage and boldness and you will be successful in your goal of Stop Smoking! Do not procrastinate for procrastination is negative thinking. I say to you, **go for it with confidence so that you can Stop Smoking Now!**

Believe me, you can be a great success in any venture if you think you can. You must think constructive thoughts supported by positive action. I mentioned the *Cogito* of Rene Descartes in the first chapter of this book to illustrate the power of thought. Now here is a new slant to the *Cogito*.

I think that I have the power within me to give up smoking easily, completely, and effortlessly, therefore, I can stop smoking now!

Now think about that, articulate it by action, doing something new. Remember the fundamental principles of mind technique that I discussed in chapter one. If you truly believe that you can do it then, so be it, you can. Remember that a true belief, in the sense that I use *belief* in this book, is one that is like faith and ignites serious positive action.

3.8 Practice Sessions
How to Give Yourself a Confidence Booster
Follow the method which I have discussed above and proceed with personal instructions about what is to be done, then follow up with deep relaxation and finally the essential positive mental prompts at the moment of ultimate deep relaxation.

If you think that it is more convenient for you to listen to your positive mental prompts, then you may record them on any multi-media devise and listen to your recording regularly. Your mind will absorb it quicker because you will be listening to your own voice, the ideas become your thought bricks and the effect of listening to them is astonishingly therapeutic.

I give you a guide here. The guide is as given before, the same order but, different words, different pictures, and different imagery so you have many to choose from each of the chapters of this book. You may proceed as follows.

Instructions

To begin with, find yourself a very comfortable position, sitting or lying down and proceed as follows. Put yourself into a state of deep relaxation in accordance with the methods which I have demonstrated in this book. While remaining in this deeply relaxed state, give yourself positive mental prompts for the idea of success in your desire to stop smoking easily, completely, and effectively as follows.

Relaxation

Take a long, slow, deep breath through your diaphragm and hold it to a mental count of five, or ten. Now open your mouth slowly and gently exhale all the air from your body as you allow the feeling of relaxation to spread through your body from the top of your head to the tips of your toes.

As you relax, you will think positive thoughts about success in your goal to stop smoking easily, completely, effectively, and effortlessly. Now go deeper, deeper, and deeper into peace, going into a higher state of consciousness in relation to your desire to stop smoking completely, feeling completely fresh from the inside, feeling good and looking good.

Positive Mental Prompts

From this moment, onwards you will think positive thoughts so that positive feelings will flow to you in relation to success in your desire to stop smoking, easily completely and effectively. You have let go your tense hold on negative thoughts and negative emotions. Now you must let go everything that went on in the past that was unsuccessful in your attempts to stop smoking or in any area of your life. You are concentrating on success now because success is what you want.

The past will cease to bother you from now because you have great confidence in yourself and in your plans to stop smoking now! You have planned the way you want to live your life. Your life will be free from smoking from now onwards and the future will be exactly what you want it to be, it will be according to your plans.

You will stop smoking, easily, completely, and effectively, you will be fit, healthy and energetic because you have stopped smoking. You will look good and feel great from now onwards. Your breath will be clean and fresh because you have eliminated the nicotine, tar, and poison of cigarette smoke.

You have eliminated restrictive mental frameworks relating to the idea of success in your desire to stop smoking easily, completely, and effectively. You have let go mistaken beliefs relating to what you want to achieve so your success in your desire to stop smoking will come to you through your positive thoughts and attitudes.

Your mind is now clearly attuned to success in your chosen goal so your goal to stop smoking will be achieved easily, completely, effectively, and effortlessly. You are genuinely and seriously concerned with success. You will achieve success because you are a determined person.

You are firm and resolute in your search for success. You will derive great satisfaction from your plans to stop smoking easily, completely, effectively, and effortlessly.

Day by day in every way from now onwards, as you relax you will find that the road to success in your goal to stop smoking is clearly sign-posted for you and you will get there and walk on the road of success, where you truly belong. You know that success in your plans to stop smoking easily, completely, and effectively is possible for you because everything is possible with the power of your mind.

Everyday in every way you will become more and more relaxed in whatever you do. You will find that relaxation will give you the peace of mind and the inner tranquillity which will enable you to develop much more confidence in yourself. You will become much more confident in yourself. You will become much more confident your ability to do the things that matter in your life. You will also be confident in doing the things that will bring greater success to you in your desire to stop smoking easily, completely, and effectively.

From this moment, onwards you will be self-reliant. You are now full of independence and you have a determination to achieve success in your goal to stop smoking now. You have a great inner courage to succeed. Feel it now. Listen to your inner self. Everyday in every way from this moment onwards you will become more and more self confident as each day brings success to you in whatever you do from day to day.

You will begin now to project a new, positive, self image and you will be successful. As success begins to take over in your life, you will find that you will be happier and contented with what you are doing, much more cheerful and much more optimistic about your future in relation to your goal to stop smoking now. You will use your mind much more clearly and effectively as you come to appreciate the enormous power of your mind to bring success into your life. You will know it to be true that the magic of success is truly within you.

You can now make decisions easily, readily, and correctly. As the decisions that you make bring successes into your life with each passing day, you will find that your life is filled with rich and excitingly rewarding things to do to bring you further success, joy and happiness. So, go for it now with confidence and you will always be successful in anything that you do as you stop smoking successfully easily, completely, and effectively.

3.9 Affirmations to Bring the Results that You Desire
Affirmations to help you to stop smoking now
Affirmations have truly magical powers which bring desired results to genuine seekers of success. I have been stating the general rule with affirmations all through this book.

The rule is that you must always affirm what you want to achieve, not the negation of what you want to achieve. You must not affirm the things, conditions or the state of affairs which you do not require in your life. In brief, you must always affirm your wishes, desires, intentions, goals, etc and not the negation of your desire or intention.

There is a popular statement that people make generally with good intentions. This statement is that, "Nothing is Impossible". This functions as an affirmation for those making it. However, following our rules of affirmation here, the popular statement is a negative affirmation. It is dealing with "Nothing" and "Impossible".

If there is genuine intention in your affirmation, you will want your affirmation to relate to something which has a possibility of fulfilment. This is why you are making the affirmation.

However, you will notice that "Nothing" and "Impossible" are not the terms which are appropriate for the description of what you wish to achieve or accomplish. Under such circumstances, the appropriate affirmation should be that, "Everything is Possible".

Here you are dealing with possibilities. Any goal, wishes, or desires that you might wish to accomplish is something which is within the realm of possibilities and it is entailed by everything.

You must never deal with the negation of your intentions, just say what you want, not the negation of what you want. Here are more illustrations to serve as further guides as follows.

I am a non-smoker.
I am a confident, positive, and very optimistic person.
I am happy, cheerful, and always relaxed.

The above statements are positive affirmations of the qualities and moods you wish to retain in your life. In contrast to the above, examine the following statement.

I do not want to be unhappy and I am not tense and not angry.

You must always guard against the temptation to make such statement as the one above because it is the affirmation of the negative traits which you should always avoid. The general rule is to concentrate on what you want and affirm it. In the above statement, the emphasis is on *unhappy, tense,* and *angry.*

These are the traits you do not want but they are the ones that the unconscious mind has received. For this reason, those traits will, unfortunately, underline your mood! If you are uncertain about this you can refer to my discussion of the power of the unconscious mind in chapter one.

Affirmations are very powerful thought bricks of the mind. They work because they follow the fundamental principles of mind techniques which I discussed in chapter one. They are part of the thought bricks which form the structures of the mind castle which you wish to build. This means that what you affirm is what you get. The statement that forms your affirmation is your declaration, something which you have endorsed or ratified. This is what it means to *affirm* something.

Affirmation of Action

This is concerned with a planned positive action which will result in the achievement of a desired goal. An individual may have difficulty in giving up smoking or in performing other chosen tasks. In such situations, the appropriate affirmations which the individual should make would be made as follows.

I will stop smoking now easily, completely, and effectively.
I will perform simple physical exercises every day, for my health and fitness.
I will always make determined and resolute plans from now onwards.
I will always finish whatever I start.
The achievement of my goal is guaranteed by my positive actions.
Whenever I plan to do something, I see it to the end.
From this moment onwards, I will always work hard to maintain my health.
I will stop smoking now to regain my strength and stamina!

In the above affirmations, you are making positive statements, you are affirming your determination to finish the work that you have started, stop smoking now, affirming the result of your determination, that is, that you will finish what you have started by seeing things to the end and you are affirming that you will stop smoking now! What happens is that if you have made the affirmation with genuine feelings, the positive nature of the affirmation will stir your mind to positive action which is expressed in your continued positive thoughts and positive attitudes towards your goal to maintain your health or stop smoking whichever is applicable.

With respect to stop smoking, the result of the combined mental operations is that you will be able to stop smoking easily, completely, and effectively. Remember the principles of mind power, if you think it and believe it, you will get it because the thought and the belief will provoke you to effective positive action. This is the essence of my powerful statements in the introductory chapter where I said that you will get what you want because what you want is what you get. The emphasis is on the verbs, the action words, *want* and *get*.

Affirmation of Thought Bricks

This is mental affirmation. In this affirmation, you use thought bricks with which to construct your mind castles. You make such affirmations mentally to yourself. For example, in my illustration in the last section, *the 60 Cigarettes a Day Smoker* may affirm the statements of plans 1 and 2 constantly and then back up the mental affirmation with positive action to improve his physical strength and appearance. On the other hand, the individual may affirm the idea of success and the result of success as follows

I am always in control of my life.
I know what I want and how to get it.
I will get what I am looking for because what I am looking for is what I want.
I will stop smoking because I want to be a non-smoker.
I will stop smoking now because I have a great concern for my health.
I will stop smoking easily, completely, effectively, and effortlessly.

If this affirmation is made constantly, it will be retained in the unconscious mind and this will lead to new ways for achieving success in the individual's life and ways of achieving the goal to stop smoking easily, completely, effectively, and effortlessly.

Written Affirmations

This can take the form of a written out positive plan of what the individual wishes to accomplish in his life. Remember that I mentioned in the last chapter that a goal that is well formulated must be kept constantly in mind. The best way to do this is to affirm the goal constantly. This makes the goal easily amenable to fulfilment.

Take care and affirm confidently and you will be successful in your goal. Remember the five fundamental principles which I discussed in chapter one and apply those principles in everything you do from day to day. I expect that from this moment onwards, you will be looking good and feeling good, always.

CHAPTER FOUR: RECAPITULATION OF SOME ESSENTIAL POINTS

As a follow up, to my discussions of affirmations and a fitting conclusion to this book, I wish to discuss here the essential final points which you must try to remember as these will help you to build your confidence and make you more determined to stop smoking now!

4.1 The Logic of Numbers

Always remember that the logic of numbers helps to determine your success in whatever you do. The more times you practise all the exercises in this book the better chance you will have of achieving your objective to stop smoking. Remember the saying, *practise makes perfect*. You will become perfect in whatever you do the more times you practise on it. Here is an illustration with practical affairs as a guide for you as follows.

Suppose that you are an athlete and you want to improve your personal best (PB) performance on your event. The logic of numbers stipulates that the more times your practise, the better you become in your event. Also, in the same way, let us suppose that you are looking for a job. The logic of numbers stipulates that if you send out 100 job applications every week your chance of being invited for an interview would be much better than if you send out one job application every week

Remember the saying, *If, at first, you don't succeed, try, try, try again.* This saying implicates the logic of numbers as it is a statement of determined achievers. Persistence and perseverance are an application of the logic of numbers. An individual must be persistent in what he or she does because it shows a dogged determination to succeed in a chosen objective. The principle of the logic of numbers is a doctrine for determined achievers. The principle is easy to understand and simple to apply in your daily routines.

The principle of the logic of numbers is implicated in a general way in the fundamental principles of thought bricks which I discussed in the first part of this book. When you have positive thoughts about your plans and your objective to stop smoking and practise the mental exercises in this book, you will find that you will stop smoking now, easily, completely, and effortlessly.

4.2 The Magic of Success

Always remember that the thought bricks for success in any venture are constructed in the mind. In any situation, if you think you can, you are already on your way to the winning post. It is all in the state of the mind.

Your success in anything you do begins in your mind. This is the essence of the fundamental principles of the mind technique which I discussed in chapter one. The mind is the magic power that a person can use to achieve great success in whatever he or she does.

Thus, you must always attune your mind to success and you will be successful in whatever you do. Remember that *the magic of success is truly within you.* It is within your mind. Apply the magic now in your attempt to stop smoking and you will notice that you will stop smoking now easily, completely, and effortlessly, almost magically.

4.3 The Pitfalls of Negative Prompts

Always think positive thoughts about your goals. When you give suggestions to yourself or whenever you make affirmations about your goal to stop smoking, use positive words that enhance your desire. Always affirm your objectives or whatever you wish to achieve and avoid the temptation to use negative expressions in talking about your goal. Examine the following illustrations.

(a) I will not fail to stop smoking.
(b) During tomorrow's meeting, I will not be tired and I will not be sleepy.

You will notice that (a) and (b) above are very negative expressions in terms of what the individual wishes to accomplish. They are about what you will not do and (a) is already talking about failure before the event. In consideration of what you want to achieve the correct, positive, expression should be as follows.

(c) I will be successful in my goal to stop smoking easily, completely, effectively, and effortlessly.
(d) During tomorrow's meeting, I will be wide awake and alert.

Notice that (c) and (d) above show more determination than (a) and (b). When your suggestions, affirmations or mental prompts are made in an emphatic way as (c) and (d) they become more effective for you. For more discussions on the pitfalls of negative prompts refer to my book, *Mind Castles* (2002).

4.4 Action is the Route to Change

Action is necessary to bring about the changes that you require. If you fail to act then no changes will be made to the existing situation and the lack of change will be due to your lack of action. If you have a genuine, serious, intention to stop smoking then you owe it to yourself to perform all the necessary actions as advised in this book. Remember the principles of the action plan which I drew out for the *60 Cigarettes a Day Smoker* in chapter two above and draw out a similar plan of action to suit your purpose.

4.5 Belief is the Ultimate

Belief is an essential ingredient in a recipe for success in anything you do. You can be a great success in any venture if you believe that you can. Remember that no one is ready for success in any venture until he or she believes that he or she can be successful in it.

Remember also that belief is the opposite of doubt. When you have belief, you always pursue your goal with a determination to attain the goal. Your belief is a thought brick. You must think constructive thoughts supported by positive actions that affirm your belief. For the purpose of your goal to stop smoking, a statement of belief can be expressed as follows.

- ❖ *I have the power to stop smoking now because I know that my success is guaranteed by my belief.*
- ❖ *I can get whatever I am looking for because I believe that I can.*
- ❖ *I can stop smoking now easily, completely, effectively, and effortlessly because I believe that I can.*

When you can make such statements as the above in relation to your goals and aspirations, you will know for certain that you are on the way to achieving your objective. I am concerned here with genuine belief so the above statements are not meant to be mere verbal utterances. Notice that in the above statements, the action words, that is, the words constituting the actions, such as *stop, get* are all affirmed by the belief.

For your goal to stop smoking, it is important that you have your belief as a mental theory of success. This ensures that when you genuinely believe that you can stop smoking now, your belief guarantees your success in your goal to stop smoking because your belief has been retained in the unconscious mind as a positive and highly effective thought brick. This means that, for you, success in your goal to stop smoking exists as a thought process in your mind and that you are aware of this.

You can see clearly from what I have stated variously here, that when such thought process has taken hold in the unconscious mind, the individual's attitude towards success in the goal to stop smoking, or in any venture, betrays the existence of positive thoughts about your goal to stop smoking and about success in general.

When you experience such a situation you know that you will always be successful with your goal because your positive attitude towards your goal clearly manifests your confidence and your success is guaranteed by your belief which induces your positive action. Your belief is a spur to a positive action. It gives momentum to the action which you must take to accomplish your goal.

In this way, the thought brick which entails your goal is always with you, always in your mind. As you know from my discussions about goals, in this book, to achieve success with your goal to stop smoking, the goal must be kept constantly in your mind at all times otherwise you may run the risk of supplanting it with some other wish or desire. Refer to my discussions about goals in chapter two and my discussions about the fundamental principles of the mind technique in chapter one.

Remember that your success in your goal or venture is assured by your positive action to attain the goal. In coming this far to the last chapter of the book, you have already made a positive action. Remember that your journey to the world of positive possibilities, at the beginning of this book, helps to set the psychical system in motion to enable you to feel relaxed always.

Now, try to practise the knowledge that you have gained from this book. Repeat the journey whenever it is necessary for you to do so and use the journey to achieve any other goals that you may have. Perform the exercises which are given in this book to attain a deeply relaxed mind and body so that you will be always successful in what you do. Congratulations to you for coming to the end of the book. Well done.

REFERENCES

The references given below are of books which are mentioned in the text

Descartes, Rene. 1641 *Meditations on First Philosophy*

Descartes, Rene. 1637 *Discourse on Method*

Freud, Sigmund. 1916-1917: Introductory Lectures on Psychoanalysis PFL Vol 1

Jung, Carl Gustav. *Collected Works Volume 8*

Maurice-Nneke, Antony. 2003. *The Psychodynamics of The Unconscious.* Intapsy Publications, London

Maurice-Nneke, Antony. 2002. *Mind Castles*. Intapsy Publications. London

Shakespeare, William. *Hamlet*